# Understanding the Role of the Immune System in Improving Tissue Regeneration

PROCEEDINGS OF A WORKSHOP

Anna Nicholson, Samantha N. Schumm, and Sarah H. Beachy,
*Rapporteurs*

Forum on Regenerative Medicine

Board on Health Sciences Policy

Health and Medicine Division

*The National Academies of*
SCIENCES • ENGINEERING • MEDICINE

THE NATIONAL ACADEMIES PRESS
*Washington, DC*
www.nap.edu

THE NATIONAL ACADEMIES PRESS    500 Fifth Street, NW    Washington, DC 20001

This activity was supported by contracts between the National Academy of Sciences and Advanced Regenerative Manufacturing Institute; Akron Biotech; Alliance for Regenerative Medicine; American Society of Gene & Cell Therapy; Burroughs Wellcome Fund (Grant No. 1021433); California Institute for Regenerative Medicine; Centre for Commercialization of Regenerative Medicine; Department of Veterans Affairs (Contract No. 36C24E21C0011; IFCAP-PO # 127-D12013); Food and Drug Administration: Center for Biologics Evaluation and Research (Grant No. 5R13FD006614-03); International Society for Cellular Therapy; International Society for Stem Cell Research; Johnson & Johnson; National Institute of Standards and Technology; National Institutes of Health: National Center for Advancing Translational Sciences; National Eye Institute; National Heart, Lung, and Blood Institute; National Institute on Aging; National Institute of Biomedical Imaging and Bioengineering; National Institute of Dental and Craniofacial Research; National Institute of Diabetes and Digestive and Kidney Diseases; National Institute of Neurological Disorders and Stroke (Contract No. HHSN263201800029I; Order No. 75N98019F00847; Mod. P00002); The New York Stem Cell Foundation; and United Therapeutics Corporation (No. 4500035476). Any opinions, findings, conclusions, or recommendations expressed in this publication do not necessarily reflect the views of any organization or agency that provided support for the project.

International Standard Book Number-13: 978-0-309-68817-8
International Standard Book Number-10: 0-309-68817-5
Digital Object Identifier: https://doi.org/10.17226/26551

Additional copies of this report are available for sale from the National Academies Press, 500 Fifth Street, NW, Keck 360, Washington, DC 20001; (800) 624-6242 or (202) 334-3313; http://www.nap.edu.

Copyright 2022 by the National Academy of Sciences. All rights reserved.

Printed in the United States of America

Suggested citation: National Academies of Sciences, Engineering, and Medicine. 2022. *Understanding the role of the immune system in improving tissue regeneration: Proceedings of a workshop*. Washington, DC: The National Academies Press. https://doi.org/10.17226/26551.

*The National Academies of*
SCIENCES · ENGINEERING · MEDICINE

The **National Academy of Sciences** was established in 1863 by an Act of Congress, signed by President Lincoln, as a private, nongovernmental institution to advise the nation on issues related to science and technology. Members are elected by their peers for outstanding contributions to research. Dr. Marcia McNutt is president.

The **National Academy of Engineering** was established in 1964 under the charter of the National Academy of Sciences to bring the practices of engineering to advising the nation. Members are elected by their peers for extraordinary contributions to engineering. Dr. John L. Anderson is president.

The **National Academy of Medicine** (formerly the Institute of Medicine) was established in 1970 under the charter of the National Academy of Sciences to advise the nation on medical and health issues. Members are elected by their peers for distinguished contributions to medicine and health. Dr. Victor J. Dzau is president.

The three Academies work together as the **National Academies of Sciences, Engineering, and Medicine** to provide independent, objective analysis and advice to the nation and conduct other activities to solve complex problems and inform public policy decisions. The National Academies also encourage education and research, recognize outstanding contributions to knowledge, and increase public understanding in matters of science, engineering, and medicine.

Learn more about the National Academies of Sciences, Engineering, and Medicine at **www.nationalacademies.org**.

*The National Academies of*
SCIENCES • ENGINEERING • MEDICINE

**Consensus Study Reports** published by the National Academies of Sciences, Engineering, and Medicine document the evidence-based consensus on the study's statement of task by an authoring committee of experts. Reports typically include findings, conclusions, and recommendations based on information gathered by the committee and the committee's deliberations. Each report has been subjected to a rigorous and independent peer-review process and it represents the position of the National Academies on the statement of task.

**Proceedings** published by the National Academies of Sciences, Engineering, and Medicine chronicle the presentations and discussions at a workshop, symposium, or other event convened by the National Academies. The statements and opinions contained in proceedings are those of the participants and are not endorsed by other participants, the planning committee, or the National Academies.

For information about other products and activities of the National Academies, please visit www.nationalacademies.org/about/whatwedo.

## PLANNING COMMITTEE ON UNDERSTANDING THE ROLE OF THE IMMUNE SYSTEM IN IMPROVING TISSUE REGENERATION[1]

**NADYA LUMELSKY** (*Co-Chair*), Chief, Integrative Biology and Infectious Diseases Branch; Director, Tissue Engineering and Regenerative Medicine Program, National Institute of Dental and Craniofacial Research, National Institutes of Health
**KIMBERLEE POTTER** (*Co-Chair*), Scientific Program Manager, Biomedical Laboratory R&D Service, Office of Research & Development, Department of Veterans Affairs
**STEVEN BECKER**, Associate Director, Office of Regenerative Medicine, National Eye Institute, National Institutes of Health (*at the time the committee was formed*)
**JENNIFER ELISSEEFF**, Jules Stein Professor, Morton Goldberg Professor; Director, Translational Tissue Engineering Center, Johns Hopkins University
**SADIK KASSIM**, Chief Technology Officer, Vor Biopharma
**CANDACE KERR**, Program Officer, Division of Aging Biology, National Institute on Aging, National Institutes of Health
**CATO LAURENCIN**, University Professor, Albert and Wilda Van Dusen Distinguished Professor; Director, The Raymond and Beverly Sackler Center for Biomedical, Biological, Physical, and Engineering Sciences; Chief Executive Officer, Connecticut Convergence Institute for Translation in Regenerative Engineering, University of Connecticut
**RICHARD MCFARLAND**, Chief Regulatory Officer, Advanced Regenerative Manufacturing Institute
**RACHEL SALZMAN**, Chair, Government Relations Committee, American Society of Gene and Cell Therapy
**SOHEL TALIB**, Senior Science Officer and Director of Therapeutics, California Institute for Regenerative Medicine
**DANIEL WEISS**, Chief Scientific Officer, International Society for Cell & Gene Therapy; Professor, University of Vermont

*Forum on Regenerative Medicine Staff*

**SARAH H. BEACHY**, Senior Program Officer and Forum Director
**SIOBHAN ADDIE**, Program Officer (*until August 2021*)
**MEREDITH HACKMANN**, Associate Program Officer

---

[1] The National Academies of Sciences, Engineering, and Medicine's planning committees are solely responsible for organizing the workshop, identifying topics, and choosing speakers. The responsibility for the published Proceedings of a Workshop rests with the workshop rapporteurs and the institution.

**SAMANTHA SCHUMM,** Associate Program Officer (*from September 2021*)
**LYDIA TEFERRA,** Research Assistant

*Board on Health Sciences Policy Staff*

**BRIDGET BOREL,** Program Coordinator
**ANDREW M. POPE,** Senior Board Director

# FORUM ON REGENERATIVE MEDICINE[1]

**TIM COETZEE** (*Co-Chair*), Chief Advocacy, Services, and Science Officer, National Multiple Sclerosis Society
**KATHERINE TSOKAS** (*Co-Chair*), Vice President, Regulatory, Quality, Risk Management and Drug Safety, Janssen Inc. Canada
**SANGEETA BHATIA,** John J. and Dorothy Wilson Professor, Institute for Medical Engineering and Science, Electrical Engineering and Computer Science, Massachusetts Institute of Technology
**PHILIP JOHN BROOKS,** Program Director, Office of Rare Disease Research, National Center for Advancing Translational Sciences, National Institutes of Health
**GEORGE Q. DALEY,** Director, Stem Cell Transplantation Program, Boston Children's Hospital and Dana-Farber Cancer Institute; Dean, Harvard Medical School
**RENA D'SOUZA** (*from June 2021*), Director, National Institute of Dental and Craniofacial Research, National Institutes of Health
**LAWRENCE GOLDSTEIN,** Distinguished Professor, Department of Cellular and Molecular Medicine, Department of Neurosciences; Director, University of California, San Diego Stem Cell Program; Scientific Director, Sanford Consortium for Regenerative Medicine; Director, Sanford Stem Cell Clinical Center, University of California, San Diego School of Medicine
**CANDACE KERR,** Program Officer, Stem Cell Program, Aging Physiology Branch Division of Aging Biology, National Institute on Aging, National Institutes of Health
**ROBERT S. LANGER,** David H. Koch Institute Professor, Massachusetts Institute of Technology
**CATO T. LAURENCIN,** University Professor, Albert and Wilda Van Dusen Distinguished Professor of Orthopaedic Surgery, Professor of Chemical, Materials Science, and Biomedical Engineering; Director, The Raymond and Beverly Sackler Center for Biomedical, Biological, Physical, and Engineering Sciences; Chief Executive Officer, Connecticut Convergence Institute for Translation in Regenerative Engineering, University of Connecticut
**TIMOTHY LAVAUTE,** Program Director, Division of Neuroscience, National Institute of Neurological Disease and Stroke, National Institutes of Health

---

[1] The National Academies of Sciences, Engineering, and Medicine's forums and roundtables do not issue, review, or approve individual documents. The responsibility for the published Proceedings of a Workshop rests with the workshop rapporteurs and the institution.

**TERRY MAGNUSON,** Sarah Graham Kenan Professor, Vice Chancellor for Research, University of North Carolina at Chapel Hill
**MICHAEL MAY,** President and Chief Executive Officer, Centre for Commercialization of Regenerative Medicine
**RICHARD McFARLAND,** Chief Regulatory Officer, Advanced Regenerative Manufacturing Institute
**JACK T. MOSHER,** Senior Manager, Scientific Affairs, International Society for Stem Cell Research
**AMY PATTERSON,** Chief Science Advisor and Director of Scientific Research Programs, National Heart, Lung, and Blood Institute, National Institutes of Health
**DUANQING PEI,** Director General, Guangzhou Institutes of Biomedicine and Health, Chinese Academy of Sciences
**THOMAS PETERSEN,** Vice President, Regenerative Medicine, United Therapeutics Corporation
**ANNE PLANT,** NIST Fellow, National Institute of Standards and Technology
**KIMBERLEE POTTER,** Scientific Program Manager, Biomedical Laboratory R&D Service, Office of Research and Development, Department of Veterans Affairs
**DAVID RAMPULLA,** Director, Division of Discovery Science & Technology, National Institute of Biomedical Imaging and Bioengineering, National Institutes of Health
**DEREK ROBERTSON,** Co-Founder and President, Maryland Sickle Cell Disease Association
**KELLY ROSE,** Program Officer, Burroughs Wellcome Fund
**KRISHNENDU ROY,** Robert A. Milton Chair and Professor in Biomedical Engineering; Technical Lead, National Cell Manufacturing Consortium; Director, Marcus Center for Therapeutic Cell Characterization and Manufacturing, Georgia Institute of Technology
**KRISHANU SAHA,** Associate Professor and Retina Research Foundation Kathryn and Latimer Murfee Chair, Department of Biomedical Engineering, University of Wisconsin–Madison
**RACHEL SALZMAN,** Chair, Government Relations Committee, American Society of Gene and Cell Therapy
**IVONNE SCHULMAN,** Program Director, National Institute of Diabetes and Digestive and Kidney Diseases, National Institutes of Health
**JAY P. SIEGEL,** (retired) Chief Biotechnology Officer and Head, Scientific Strategy and Policy, Johnson & Johnson
**LANA SKIRBOLL,** Vice President, Science Policy, Sanofi
**SUSAN L. SOLOMAN,** Founder and Chief Executive Officer, New York Stem Cell Foundation

**MARTHA SOMERMAN** (*until June 2021*), Director, National Institute of Dental and Craniofacial Research, National Institutes of Health
**MICHAEL STEINMETZ,** Director, Division of Extramural Science Programs, National Eye Institute, National Institutes of Health
**SOHEL TALIB,** Senior Science Officer and Director of Therapeutics, California Institute for Regenerative Medicine
**DANIEL WEISS,** Chief Scientific Officer, International Society for Cell & Gene Therapy
**MICHAEL WERNER,** Co-Founder and Senior Policy Counsel, Alliance for Regenerative Medicine
**CELIA WITTEN,** Deputy Director, Center for Biologics Evaluation and Research, U.S. Food and Drug Administration
**CLAUDIA ZYLBERBERG,** Founder and Chief Executive Officer, Akron Biotech

*Forum on Regenerative Medicine Staff*

**SARAH H. BEACHY,** Senior Program Officer and Forum Director
**SIOBHAN ADDIE,** Program Officer (*until August 2021*)
**MEREDITH HACKMANN,** Associate Program Officer
**SAMANTHA SCHUMM,** Associate Program Officer (*from September 2021*)
**LYDIA TEFERRA,** Research Assistant

*Board on Health Sciences Policy Staff*

**BRIDGET BOREL,** Program Coordinator
**ANDREW M. POPE,** Senior Board Director

# Reviewers

This Proceedings of a Workshop was reviewed in draft form by individuals chosen for their diverse perspectives and technical expertise. The purpose of this independent review is to provide candid and critical comments that will assist the National Academies of Sciences, Engineering, and Medicine in making each published proceedings as sound as possible and to ensure that it meets the institutional standards for quality, objectivity, evidence, and responsiveness to the charge. The review comments and draft manuscript remain confidential to protect the integrity of the process.

We thank the following individuals for their review of this proceedings:

**STEVEN BECKER,** National Cancer Institute
**ERIKA MOORE,** University of Florida

Although the reviewers listed above provided many constructive comments and suggestions, they were not asked to endorse the content of the proceedings nor did they see the final draft before its release. The review of this proceedings was overseen by **LESLIE Z. BENET,** University of California, San Francisco. He was responsible for making certain that an independent examination of this proceedings was carried out in accordance with standards of the National Academies and that all review comments were carefully considered. Responsibility for the final content rests entirely with the rapporteurs and the National Academies.

We also thank staff member Julie Schuck for reading and providing helpful comments on this manuscript.

# Acknowledgments

The support of the sponsors of the Forum on Regenerative Medicine was crucial to the planning and conduct of the workshop, Understanding the Role of the Immune System in Improving Tissue Regeneration, and for the development of this Proceedings of a Workshop. Federal sponsors were the Department of Veterans Affairs; U.S. Food and Drug Administration: Center for Biologics Evaluation and Research; National Institute of Standards and Technology; National Institutes of Health: National Center for Advancing Translational Sciences; National Eye Institute; National Heart, Lung, and Blood Institute; National Institute on Aging; National Institute of Biomedical Imaging and Bioengineering; National Institute of Dental and Craniofacial Research; National Institute of Diabetes and Digestive and Kidney Diseases; and National Institute of Neurological Disorders and Stroke. Nonfederal sponsorship was provided by Advanced Regenerative Manufacturing Institute; Akron Biotech; Alliance for Regenerative Medicine; American Society of Gene & Cell Therapy; Burroughs Wellcome Fund; California Institute for Regenerative Medicine; Centre for Commercialization of Regenerative Medicine; International Society for Cellular Therapy; International Society for Stem Cell Research; Johnson & Johnson; The New York Stem Cell Foundation; and United Therapeutics Corporation.

The Forum on Regenerative Medicine wishes to express gratitude to the expert speakers who examined how modulation of the patient immune system and regenerative medicine products can improve the clinical outcomes of tissue repair and regeneration in patients. The Forum also wishes to thank the members of the planning committee for their work in developing an excellent workshop agenda. The project director would like to thank the project staff who worked diligently to develop both the workshop and the resulting Proceedings of a Workshop.

# Contents

BOXES, FIGURES, AND TABLE     xix
ACRONYMS AND ABBREVIATIONS     xxi

1    INTRODUCTION     1
Opening Remarks, 3
Organization of the Proceedings, 5

2    TISSUE HOMEOSTASIS, INFLAMMATION, AND REPAIR     7
Tissue Homeostasis, 8
Common Features of Tissue Organization, 8
Tissue Organization and Composition, 9
Cellular Division of Labor, 10
Minimal Tissue Units and Growth Factor Production, 10
Tissue or Organ Size Control, 13
Tissue Repair and Regeneration, 14

3    LESSONS LEARNED FROM IMMUNE TOLERANCE
AND GRAFT ACCEPTANCE     15
The Microbiome and Immune Tolerance: Lessons from
    Allogeneic Hematopoietic Cell Transplantation, 16
Immune Tolerance and Graft Acceptance: Lessons from
    Transplant Immunology, 21
Discussion, 26

4  **ENGINEERING OF ALLOGENEIC DONOR CELLS FOR ACCEPTANCE BY THE HOST'S IMMUNE SYSTEM**  33
   Mesenchymal Stromal Cells in Immunomodulatory Therapies, 34
   Protecting Transplanted Cells from Immune Rejection, 37
   Off-the-Shelf Engineered iPSC-Derived Natural Killer and T Cells for the Treatment of Cancer, 43
   Discussion, 47

5  **ENDOGENOUS REGENERATION AND THE ROLE OF THE LOCAL ENVIRONMENT IN REPAIR**  53
   Reversing Aging: Pro-Inflammatory Metabolite Prostaglandin E2 Augments Muscle Regeneration, 54
   Biomaterials for Modeling Immune Mediation in Wound Healing, 59
   Endogenous Pro-Resolution and Pro-Regenerative Mechanisms in Periodontal Tissue, 63
   Discussion, 66

6  **MODULATING THE HOST IMMUNE SYSTEM TO CREATE A PRO-REGENERATIVE ENVIRONMENT**  73
   Cellular Senescence, Senolytics, and Organ Regeneration and Transplantation, 74
   Mapping the Immune and Tissue Environment in Healing and Non-healing Wounds, 79
   Resolution of Acute Inflammation Stimulates Tissue Regeneration, 85
   Discussion, 89

7  **TOOLS AND PRECLINICAL MODELS FOR MONITORING AND OPTIMIZING THE HOST'S PRO-REGENERATIVE ENVIRONMENT**  95
   Tools for Immune Profiling and Monitoring, 96
   Engineered Immunity as a Model for Regenerative Medicine, 100
   Basic Immunology to Guide Regenerative Therapeutic Design, 104
   Discussion, 108

8  **HARNESSING THE IMMUNE SYSTEM TO IMPROVE PATIENT OUTCOMES**  113
   Final Panel Discussion, 114
   Reflections on the Workshop, 120

**REFERENCES** 127

**APPENDIXES**
A  WORKSHOP AGENDA 141
B  SPEAKER BIOGRAPHICAL SKETCHES 151
C  STATEMENT OF TASK 163

# Boxes, Figures, and Table

## BOXES

1-1  Workshop Statement of Task, 3

4-1  Advantages of Hypoimmune Cell Products, 40

5-1  Key Research Findings on the Role of Prostaglandin Signaling in Muscle Function, 59

6-1  Fundamental Aging Mechanisms and Phenotypes, 75

7-1  Impacts of CD19 CAR Therapy, 102

8-1  Ideas about the Future of Regenerative Medicine with Regard to the Immune System as Shared by Individual Presenters, 122

## FIGURES

2-1  Three types of cellular division of labor, 11
2-2  Macrophage-fibroblast two-cell circuit, 13

3-1  Microbiome and antibiotic states and clinical risk of graft-versus-host disease, 20

4-1 Overview of regenerative stem cell therapy, 38
4-2 Adaptive and innate immune responses to allogeneic cells, 41
4-3 Platform for mass production of induced pluripotent stem cell products, 45

5-1 Immune response to pro-healing versus pro-fibrotic biomaterials implanted in breast tissue, 62

6-1 Foundations of regenerative immunology, 81
6-2 Endogenous control mechanisms in resolution of inflammation, 86

## TABLE

2-1 Tissue Homeostasis, 9

# Acronyms and Abbreviations

| | |
|---|---|
| 15-PGDH | 15-hydroxyprostaglandin dehydrogenase |
| | |
| ADCC | antibody-dependent cell-mediated cytotoxicity |
| ATAC-Seq | Assay for Transposase-Accessible Chromatin with sequencing |
| AUC | area under the curve |
| | |
| Breg | regulatory B cell |
| | |
| cAMP | cyclic adenosine monophosphate |
| CAR | chimeric antigen receptor |
| CD | cluster of differentiation |
| CN | cellular neighborhood |
| CODEX | CO-Detection by indEXing |
| Co1 | cytochrome C oxidase I |
| COX | cyclooxygenase enzymes |
| CSF-1 | colony stimulating factor-1 |
| | |
| DAMP | damage-associated molecular pattern |
| DEL-1 | developmental endothelial locus-1 |
| DHEA | dehydroepiandrosterone |
| | |
| ECM | extracellular matrix |
| EGF | epidermal growth factor |

| | |
|---|---|
| EP4 | E-type prostanoid receptor 4 |
| ERK1/2 | extracellular signal-regulated protein kinase |
| ESC | embryonic stem cell |
| | |
| FAK | focal adhesion kinase |
| FDA | U.S. Food and Drug Administration |
| | |
| Gal | Galalpha1-3Galbeta1-4GlcNAc |
| GVHD | graft-versus-host disease |
| | |
| HCT | hematopoietic cell transplantation |
| HLA | human leukocyte antigen |
| HSCT | hematopoietic stem cell transplantation |
| HUVEC | human umbilical vein endothelial cell |
| | |
| ICAM-1 | intercellular adhesion molecule 1 |
| IgM | immunoglobulin M |
| IL | interleukin |
| iPSC | induced pluripotent stem cells |
| | |
| LFA-1 | lymphocyte function–associated antigen 1 |
| | |
| mAb | monoclonal antibody |
| MFGE8 | milk fat globule-EGF factor 8 protein |
| MGH | Massachusetts General Hospital |
| MHC | major histocompatibility complex |
| micro-CT | micro-computed tomography |
| miHA | minor histocompatibility antigens |
| MMP | matrix metalloproteinase |
| mRNA | messenger RNA |
| MS | multiple sclerosis |
| MSC | mesenchymal stem/stromal cell |
| mtDNA | mitochondrial DNA |
| mTOR | mammalian target of rapamycin |
| MuSC | muscle stem cell |
| MyoD | myoblast determination protein 1 |
| | |
| NF-kB | nuclear factor kappa B |
| NHP | nonhuman primate |
| NK | natural killer |
| NSAID | non-steroidal anti-inflammatory drug |

| | |
|---|---|
| P | passage |
| PAMP | pathogen-associated molecular pattern |
| PAX7 | paired box 7 |
| PCL | polycaprolactone |
| PDGF | platelet-derived growth factor |
| PD-L1 | programmed death-ligand 1 |
| PGD2 | prostaglandin D2 |
| PGE2 | prostaglandin E2 |
| PMN | polymorphonuclear neutrophil |
| PS | phosphatidylserine |
| | |
| RGD | arginine-glycine-aspartic acid |
| ROC | receiver operating characteristic |
| ROCK2 | rho-associated coiled-coil-containing protein kinase |
| RUNX2 | runt-related transcription factor 2 |
| | |
| SASP | senescent-associated secretory phenotype |
| SCAP | senescent cell anti-apoptotic pathway |
| SPM | specialized pro-resolving mediator |
| | |
| TGF-beta | transforming growth factor beta |
| Th | T helper cell |
| TLI | total lymphoid irradiation |
| TMJ | temporomandibular joint |
| TRAF3 | tumor necrosis factor receptor-associated factor 3 |
| Treg | regulatory T cell |
| | |
| uPAR | urokinase plasminogen activator receptor |
| | |
| VDJ | variable, diversity, joining |
| VEGF | vascular endothelial growth factor |

# 1

# Introduction[1]

The innate and adaptive immune systems are cornerstones of the human body's response to tissue damage and injury. The innate immune system, which is the body's nonspecific line of defense against non-self pathogens, is initially activated in response to tissue damage. As part of the healing process, acute inflammation via the innate immune system is associated with tissue repair and regeneration (Julier et al., 2017). Through the recruitment of neutrophils and macrophages, the early immune response clears cellular debris, remodels the extracellular matrix, and induces the production of high levels of cytokines (Julier et al., 2017). The adaptive immune system is subsequently activated, serving a critical role in tissue repair and regeneration through the activity of immune cells and their interactions with tissue-resident stem cells.

During normal homeostasis processes, such as cell turnover, the immune system's essential role in facilitating tissue repair and regeneration is well characterized. However, in the context of a cell-damaging event, such as injury, less is known about the specific mechanisms that activate the immune system to shift the balance toward tissue regeneration. Moreover, within the adaptive immune system, the specific molecular interactions

---

[1] The planning committee's role was limited to planning the workshop, and the Proceedings of a Workshop was prepared by the workshop rapporteurs as a factual summary of what occurred at the workshop. Statements, recommendations, and opinions expressed are those of individual presenters and participants; have not been endorsed or verified by the Health and Medicine Division of the National Academies of Sciences, Engineering, and Medicine; and should not be construed as reflecting any group consensus.

between T cells and tissue-resident stem cells—and how these two cell types contribute to overall tissue healing—have not yet been fully elucidated.

The immune system changes with advancing age. Over time, thymic atrophy can lead to a decline in adaptive immune responses and a state of chronic innate immune system activation, known as age-associated inflammation (Kasler and Verdin, 2021). This state of persistent low-grade immune activation can weaken the immune system's capacity for tissue repair and lead to the development of degenerative disease. Many regenerative medicine therapies are designed to treat age-related degenerative conditions. The development of these therapies would benefit from better understanding how the immune system is modulated during aging and how those age-related changes affect the overall coordination of endogenous tissue regeneration. A patient's immune response is also foundational to the clinical success of cell- and tissue-based regenerative medicines (Zakrzewski et al., 2014). For example, the success of allogeneic cell-based therapies can be undermined by immunological challenges, such as graft-versus-host disease and host rejection. Surmounting those challenges will require developing tolerance-inducing strategies, similar to those used to support patients receiving solid organ or hematopoietic stem cell transplants. There may be opportunities to learn from those fields how to assess a patient's immune system prior to treatment as a way to improve clinical outcomes of cell-based therapies.

Implantable, engineered biomaterials have been shown to be effective in modulating the immune system (Browne and Pandit, 2015; Sridharan et al., 2015). From a clinical perspective, however, important knowledge gaps persist at the intersection of immunology and regenerative medicine. Among the fundamental research questions to be explored are whether modulating a patient's own immune system could improve regenerative medicine outcomes and, more broadly, whether the use of regenerative medicine approaches to activate the immune response and promote tissue repair could feasibly contribute to therapeutic success.

To address these and other gaps in the understanding of promising approaches to manipulate the immune system and/or the regenerative medicine product to improve outcomes of tissue repair and regeneration in patients, the Forum on Regenerative Medicine at the National Academies of Sciences, Engineering, and Medicine convened a two-day virtual public workshop titled "Understanding the Role of the Immune System in Improving Tissue Regeneration." During the workshop, participants explored open questions about the role of the immune system in the success or failure of regenerative medicine therapies. They considered potential strategies to effectively "prepare" patients' immune systems to accept regenerative therapies and increase the likelihood of successful clinical outcomes as well as considered risks associated with modulating the immune system.

INTRODUCTION                                                                 3

Participants also reflected on lessons learned from related fields of research and clinical practice, including organ and bone marrow transplantation and age-associated inflammation. The Statement of Task for the workshop can be found in Box 1-1. A broad array of stakeholders participated in the workshop, including immunologists, cell biologists, bioengineers, industry researchers, regulatory officials, clinicians, product manufacturers, patients, and other experts.

## OPENING REMARKS

In the workshop welcome, Kathy Tsokas, vice president of Regulatory, Quality, Risk Management and Drug Safety at Janssen Inc. Canada, called for a broader conversation with the public about harnessing the

---

**BOX 1-1**
**Workshop Statement of Task**

The Forum on Regenerative Medicine will hold a public workshop to explore potential promising approaches to modulate the immune system and/or the regenerative medicine product for improving the clinical outcomes of tissue repair and regeneration in patients.

Workshop discussions may examine:

- lessons learned from other fields (e.g. organ or bone marrow transplantation) about the role of the host's immune system in accepting a graft to inform whether manipulation of a graft can impact the acceptance or rejection of it;
- topics such as potential approaches for modulating critical immune system pathways and communication mechanisms between the immune system and damaged and/or diseased tissues;
- the application of these lessons learned to the development and use of regenerative medicine products, for example:
   - what immune factors and pathways play a role in regeneration;
   - biomarkers that may be useful for assessing a patient's immune status or response to regenerative medicine therapies;
   - scaffolds, biomaterials, and other bioengineering tools that may modify immune responses; and
   - imaging technologies to leverage immune surveillance in patients and evaluation of the results of regenerative therapies.

A planning committee of the National Academies of Sciences, Engineering, and Medicine will organize the workshop, select and invite speakers and discussants, and moderate the discussions. Proceedings of the presentations and discussions at the workshop will be prepared by a designated rapporteur in accordance with institutional guidelines.

full potential of the immune system to prepare patients for more successful treatment outcomes. The discussion, she said, should center on the understanding that discoveries are for the benefit of the people who need them. In her remarks, Nadya Lumelsky, chief of the Integrative Biology and Infectious Diseases Branch and director of the Tissue Engineering and Regenerative Medicine Research Program at the National Institutes of Health's National Institute of Dental and Craniofacial Research, provided an orientation to the workshop. The goal of regenerative medicine is to repair and regenerate tissues compromised by disease, injury, or aging. This field has existed for several decades, but despite many proof-of-principle successes in animal models, relatively few therapies are currently available in clinics. This workshop was designed to address areas that could enable the accelerated translation of therapies into the clinic, with a focus on the immune system—specifically, how to leverage patients' immune systems to optimize tissue regeneration, she said.

Early attempts to regenerate tissues primarily focused on the identification and isolation of stem and progenitor cells, fueled by the idea that identifying the "right" cells would solve the problem of tissue regeneration, said Lumelsky. Although this continues to be an important area of research, it is now widely recognized that the microenvironment of tissues—often referred to as the stem cell niche—also plays a key role in the outcome of regenerative medicine therapies. Furthermore, the innate and adaptive immune systems that are part of this niche are of paramount importance. In fact, the variability in outcomes seen in the clinic with regenerative medicine therapies is often related to the patient's own immune system.

Tissue inflammation was once seen as detrimental for tissue healing and regeneration; therefore, inhibiting inflammation was believed to create a permissive environment for regeneration, Lumelsky said. However, it is now recognized that immune system inflammation is critical for effective regeneration. Productive regeneration requires certain elements of the inflammatory response, but inflammation can be problematic when it becomes chronic and initiates cyclical tissue destruction, she explained. Thus, the patterning of the immune system and controlling inflammation at the right time and place become crucial, said Lumelsky.

Lumelsky outlined two overarching themes for the workshop: (1) optimizing graft acceptance and integration of grafted cells with host tissues for cell-based regenerative therapies, and (2) optimizing the tissue microenvironment—or stem cell niche—to both promote endogenous regeneration and inhibit tissue fibrosis and scarring. In addition, participants were encouraged to discuss how to optimize therapies for translation into clinical practice. Kimberlee Potter, scientific program manager for the Biomedical Laboratory Research and Development Service at the U.S. Department of Veterans Affairs Office of Research and Development, encouraged the workshop participants, and the field at large, to center the patient in the regenerative medicine paradigm. Centering the patient in the care paradigm involves accounting for variability in patient responses to therapies. She recalled compelling stories shared by parents during a previous workshop convened by the Forum on Regenerative Medicine to explore novel clinical trial designs for gene-based therapies, in which parents described experiences their children endured with immune suppression protocols for gene-based therapies (NASEM, 2020).

Potter said that another earlier workshop, Applying Systems Thinking to Regenerative Medicine, explored critical quality attributes in cell manufacturing processes and quality-by-design manufacturing (NASEM, 2021). However, missing from the discussion was information regarding the people receiving advanced therapies and the inability to predict whether the therapy would be safe and effective. A patient-focused perspective might consider variability due to unique underlying biology and health status. With the patient at the center of the care paradigm, it is possible to develop strategies to precisely manipulate the patient's immune system to optimize graft acceptance or endogenous tissue regeneration, she added.

Keeping the patient voice at the center of the discussion was underscored by comments early in the workshop from Sherilyn George-Clinton, a leader of Multiple Sclerosis: You Are Not Alone. George-Clinton stated that she has lived with autoimmune disorders for more than 20 years. During the 11 years she has been diagnosed with multiple sclerosis, her immune system has been modulated, suppressed, and reset. She shared her enthusiasm about research to harness the immune system's powers to improve health. In this era of ultra-specialization in research, scientists should share their progress, findings, and ideas with one another, keeping patients always at the forefronts of their minds, George-Clinton remarked.

Potter also charged participants and the field to identify knowledge gaps in regenerative medicine to stimulate basic discovery science. In the current post-acute COVID-19 era, centering the immune system in discovery science can serve as a reminder that discoveries should link directly to patients receiving these therapies. Addressing knowledge gaps may involve the development of tools or preclinical models needed to mitigate risk from regenerative medicine therapies. She encouraged participants to consider how advances in fields such as organ transplantation, immunological tolerance, and wound healing can propel regenerative medicine therapies forward.

## ORGANIZATION OF THE PROCEEDINGS

This Proceedings of a Workshop summarizes the presentations and discussions that took place at the workshop on November 2 and 3, 2021.

The workshop opened with a keynote presentation on the foundational concepts of tissue homeostasis, inflammation, and repair (Chapter 2). The first session examined lessons learned about immune tolerance and graft acceptance from the field of transplant immunology with applications to regenerative medicine (Chapter 3). Speakers discussed the interaction between the microbiome and graft-versus-host disease, the potential to engineer direct differentiation in pluripotent stem cells to mesenchymal stem cells, and the value of a reverse translation approach—"from bench to bedside and back to the bench"—in developing therapies with better patient outcomes. The second session focused on efforts to engineer allogeneic donor cells for acceptance by the host's immune system (Chapter 4). Presentations and discussions explored the potential for cell-based transplantation without immunosuppression by protecting allogeneic cells from immune destruction—potentially through hypoimmune cells—and the need to identify and incorporate patient-specific biomarkers that predict outcomes to inform treatment design. The third session concentrated on endogenous regeneration and the role of the local environment in repair, with a focus on approaches that manipulate endogenous modulators of cell regeneration, cell degeneration, and aging (Chapter 5). Participants discussed how biomaterials and B cells can influence wound healing, as well as the roles of molecular mediators, prostaglandin E2 (PGE2) and developmental endothelial locus-1 (DEL-1), in healing and regenerative responses. The fourth session considered strategies to modulate the host immune system to create a pro-regenerative environment (Chapter 6). It included presentations on the applications of cellular senescence and senolytics to organ regeneration and transplantation, the use of the tissue microenvironment as an intervention target in the interdisciplinary field of regenerative immunology and immunotherapies, and the role of specialized pro-resolving mediators in the resolution of inflammation. The fifth session explored advances in developing tools and preclinical models for monitoring and optimizing the host's pro-regenerative environment (Chapter 7). Presenters described how the local biology of "cellular neighborhoods" can have prognostic and clinical value, the potential to use "living drugs" comprising engineered T cells (e.g., chimeric antigen receptor [CAR] T immunotherapies) to remove senescent cells and modulate tissue regeneration, and rational design for developing anti-fibrotic and pro-healing biomaterials. The final session featured a panel discussion on possibilities for harnessing the immune system to improve outcomes for patients (Chapter 8). The workshop closed with reflections on the future of regenerative medicine with regard to the immune system (see Box 8-1). The workshop agenda is in Appendix A. Appendix B includes speakers' biographical sketches, and Appendix C contains the approved Statement of Task for the workshop.

# 2

# Tissue Homeostasis, Inflammation, and Repair

> **Key Points Highlighted by Individual Speakers**
>
> - Compared to cellular and organismal homeostasis, tissue homeostasis is not yet well understood. (Medzhitov)
> - Cells have three division-of-labor relationships: (1) cell types perform different functions independently of one another, (2) cell types contribute to the same function, and (3) one cell type performs a function and other cell types provide support. (Medzhitov)
> - Understanding inherent tissue composition and cell interactions informs management of tissue regeneration. (Medzhitov)
> - Characterizing the rules and mechanisms that ensure production of appropriate growth factors in the correct quantity and location is key to understanding and modulating homeostasis and regenerative processes. (Medzhitov)
> - Tissues can be labile, stable, or permanent, and the characteristics of each type suggest the need for different regenerative approaches. (Medzhitov)

A keynote presentation on tissue homeostasis, inflammation, and repair was delivered by Ruslan Medzhitov, Sterling Professor of Immunobiology at Yale University School of Medicine and an investigator at Howard Hughes Medical Institute, at the beginning of the workshop. Tissue homeostasis involves the minimum cell components that constitute a tissue, a feedback circuit within the tissue, and the ways that cells within the circuit respond to environmental pressures such as available space, growth factors, cytokines, oxygen, and tension. Medzhitov reviewed the established fundamentals about these processes and highlighted gaps in our current understanding as a way to set the stage for subsequent workshop sessions on tissue regeneration.

## TISSUE HOMEOSTASIS

Much is known about cellular and organismal homeostasis, but little is understood about tissue homeostasis,[1] said Medzhitov. Cellular homeostasis involves what some biologists refer to as "cell stress responses," where cellular sensors detect levels of oxygen, glucose, protein, and other variables; when a variable changes, it initiates an appropriate adaptive response. At the systemic level, for example, oxygen stress responses to hypoxia are regulated by erythropoietin and red blood cell production, while vascularization regulates the response at the tissue level. Although angiogenesis and hypoxic response are relatively well understood, he said, most variables of tissue homeostasis are not. A number of microenvironmental variables are involved in maintaining tissue homeostasis (see Table 2-1). These include (1) oxygen and nutrients; (2) cell number and composition; (3) the composition and mechanical properties of extracellular matrix (ECM); and (4) interstitial fluid volume, pH, osmolarity, and metabolic waste products. The mechanisms that maintain these variables within tissues are unknown, with a few exceptions such as hypoxia. Medzhitov remarked that it is not the complexity of the mechanisms that impedes understanding of tissue homeostasis, but rather a lack of research in these areas.

## COMMON FEATURES OF TISSUE ORGANIZATION

Although tissue types from different organs have superficial differences in appearance, biologists have traditionally understood that all tissue types share common themes in tissue architecture and design principles. This idea is based on the understanding that a biological problem is solved by evolutionary processes, and that solution is maintained to address related problems, Medzhitov explained. For example, different tissues face similar problems, such as determining cellular composition in terms of the cell types present, their amounts and proportions, and their spatial distribution. Some cells must also be able to expand on demand, such as immune cells during an inflammatory response. He posited that early in the evolution

---

[1] Tissue homeostasis is a "collection of circuits that regulate specific variables within the tissue environment" (Meizlish et al., 2021).

**TABLE 2-1** Tissue Homeostasis

| Regulated Microenvironmental Variables | Manipulated Processes |
| --- | --- |
| Oxygen and nutrients | Local blood profusion level; angiogenesis |
| Cell number and composition | Cell proliferation; cell death; cell migration |
| ECM level, composition, and stiffness | Production and degradation of ECM components; collagen crosslinking |
| Interstitial fluids volume, pH, and osmolarity; metabolic waste products | Vascular permeability; lymphatic drainage; perfusion level; (lymph) angiogenesis; acid–base control; solute transport |

NOTE: ECM = extracellular matrix.
SOURCE: Medzhitov presentation, November 2, 2021.

of animals, a solution was developed, and in turn, all human tissues are variations on a theme related to that solution. Yet, that theme is not known. This knowledge gap limits the ability to develop rational approaches to targeting diseases at the tissue level; it is important to appreciate how little is understood at this biological level, he emphasized.

## TISSUE ORGANIZATION AND COMPOSITION

Basic tissue organization includes multiple cell types and relies upon the extracellular matrix. Tissue organization raises many questions, such as how cells "know" to exist in specific locations and what relationships there are among different cell types. Medzhitov noted that some cell types are more important than others. For example, if lymphocytes were removed from tissues, some functionalities would be lost but the overall tissue architecture would be preserved. In contrast, tissue structure is lost with the removal of fibroblasts. Thus, some cell types are more foundational than others. The question that then arises is how to define the minimal composition of tissue necessary for normal architecture, said Medzhitov. Evolutionary history can inform the answer because the simplest animals like placozoans or sponges have at least two types of cells: epithelial cells and mesenchymal cells. Together, epithelial-mesenchymal modules constitute the primordial units, or building blocks, of tissue organization.

Epithelial and mesenchymal cell types have specific relationships associated with the flow of information between them, Medzhitov explained. For example, stromal mesenchymal cells contain positional information about their location along the body's axis. They produce morphogen signals that act on epithelial cells to determine their cell fate (i.e., the different types of epithelial cells they become). This relationship between mesenchymal and epithelial cells generalizes to other cell types—that is, niche cells control the cell fate of stem cells or, in the immune system, dendritic cells control that of T cells. Furthermore, the relationship hints at the fundamental rules of tissue organization, he said. Some cells are more similar to mesenchymal cells in that they contain information, and some cells are more like epithelial or functional cell types in that they have various fate choices.

## CELLULAR DIVISION OF LABOR

Cell types also have relationships that enable them to perform necessary functions, Medzhitov noted. Cellular division of labor can be conceptualized in different ways (see Figure 2-1). Classically, the division of labor consists of two cell types that each specialize in a different function. For instance, adipocytes and osteocytes perform different functions independently of one another. Another functional relationship occurs when two cell types contribute to the same function, and both types are required to perform the function. For example, motor neurons and skeletal muscle cells are both needed to execute the function of contractility. These cell combinations are referred to as functional units.

A third form of cellular division of labor occurs when one cell type is specialized to perform a function and another cell type specializes to support the function of the first cell. For instance, a neuron is a functional cell supported by a glial Schwann cell. A Schwann cell has no functional meaning without a neuron; its meaning is predicated upon supporting a neuron. In contrast, neurons can operate without Schwann cells, and many of them do. Medzhitov added that, by analogy to client and chaperone proteins, functional and supportive cells can also be referred to as client cells and accessory cells. Applying this understanding to tissue composition underscores that some cells are more foundational than others. Some cells are functional client cells responsible for the primary function of the tissue while other cells perform supportive functions. Finally, some cells provide information relevant to fate decisions by other cells through directional signaling to those cells.

## MINIMAL TISSUE UNITS AND
## GROWTH FACTOR PRODUCTION

The minimal composition of tissues in vertebrates comprises four cell types that form "minimal tissue units," Medzhitov said. The first is responsible for the core function of the tissue and is the most common cell type of a tissue. Examples include tissue-specific cells like epithelial cells in the lung, hepatocytes in the liver, and neurons in the brain. Three other

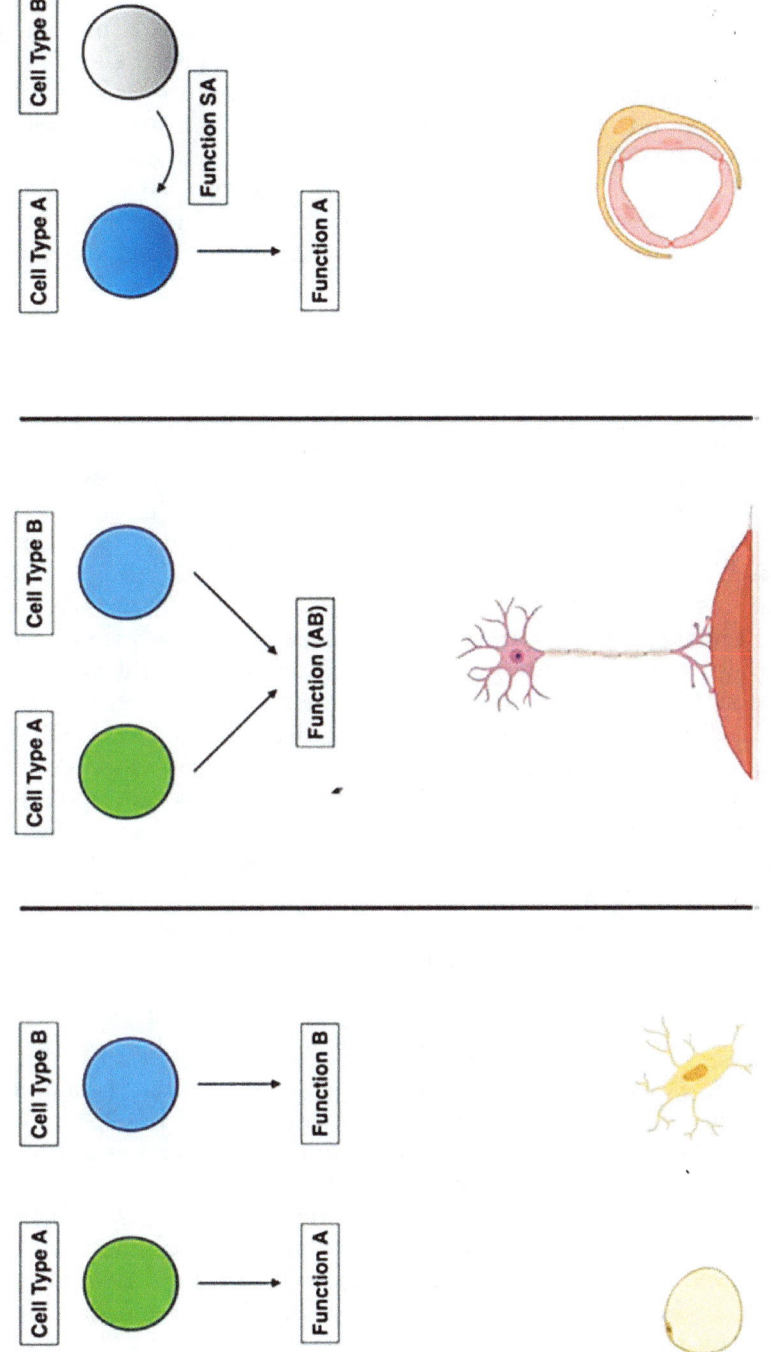

**FIGURE 2-1** Three types of cellular division of labor.
SOURCE: Medzhitov presentation, November 2, 2021.

cell types perform supportive functions: microvascular endothelial cells, fibroblast-like stromal cells, and tissue-resident macrophages. These three cell types are nearly universal in all tissues and perform supportive functions, such as delivering oxygen and nutrients, producing ECM, providing defense, and maintaining homeostasis. The primary design of a tissue consists of these four cell types, but there are exceptions; for example cartilage, he noted. Although not responsible for a primary function of the tissue, the supportive cell types are necessary for the primary cell type to perform its function optimally. The supportive cell types follow their genetically encoded instructions to support the client cell's functionality even if the client cell becomes cancerous. Therefore, the three supportive cell types are universally present in solid tumors, dutifully performing their functions despite inadvertently promoting tumor growth, Medzhitov described. This feature of supportive cells is important to consider in determining which cell categories to target for regeneration, he added.

Every normal, nontransformed cell type requires specific growth factors to survive and proliferate, and the number of cells in a given location is determined by the local availability of growth factors. Thus, the cellular composition of tissues is dictated by the local availability of lineage-specific growth factors. The question of tissue design, Medzhitov said, can be translated into a question of what controls the local provision of growth factors. For example, macrophages will not be found in tissue devoid of colony stimulating factor-1 (CSF-1), and fibroblasts make CSF-1. Similarly, macrophages and endothelial cells make platelet-derived growth factor (PDGF) to support stromal fibroblasts. The presence of cell types in the correct quantity and location depends on appropriate production of corresponding growth factors, he explained. Cells have rules and mechanisms to ensure the production of growth factors in the right amounts and locations, but these rules and mechanisms are largely unknown. Knowledge of the rules that regulate growth factor production could be applied to support the purposes of homeostasis, regeneration, or cell therapy, he suggested.

### Macrophage-Fibroblast Two-Cell Circuit

Typically, the growth factor for one cell type is produced by another, said Medzhitov. That is, cell X makes growth factor for cell Y, and the amount of growth factor determines the quantity and location of cell Y within the tissue. Generally, it is not yet understood how cells determine how much growth factor to make to ensure appropriate cell composition for the tissue. In studying macrophages and fibroblasts, Medzhitov and his colleagues found that the cell types exchange growth factors according to specific principles (Adler et al., 2018; Zhou et al., 2018). Fibroblasts produce CSF-1 for macrophages, and macrophages make PDGF for fibroblasts.

A particular regulatory circuit establishes stable provision of growth factors between macrophages and fibroblasts (see Figure 2-2). Space availability limits growth of fibroblasts while growth factor availability limits macrophages. Furthermore, this circuit design is stable to perturbations, and the concept of a minimum stable circuit is likely generalizable to other systems and cell types, including immune cells, Medzhitov explained (Zhou et al., 2018). He added that the source of growth factor for the client cell type could be regulated by a principle such as extrinsic space restriction.

## TISSUE OR ORGAN SIZE CONTROL

Medzhitov outlined two coexisting paradigms for regulating compartment (e.g., tissue or organ) size. The first paradigm centers on space availability. In this model, cells in the tissue compartment proliferate until they fill all available space, at which point proliferation ceases. The in vitro counterpart is contact inhibition. This scenario applies to some cells—such as fibroblasts and endothelial cells—but not to others, including hematopoietic cells, lymphocytes, and granulocytes. The second paradigm centers on growth factor availability and proposes that tissues locally produce appropriate amounts of growth factor. An abundance of growth factor induces cell proliferation, and if cells proliferate beyond a level sustainable by the amount of growth factor, excess cells die to reach the appropriate compartment size.

Given that fibroblasts are limited by space availability and macrophages are limited by growth factor availability, these two regulatory paradigms correspond exactly with the two cell types. Moreover, Medzhitov added,

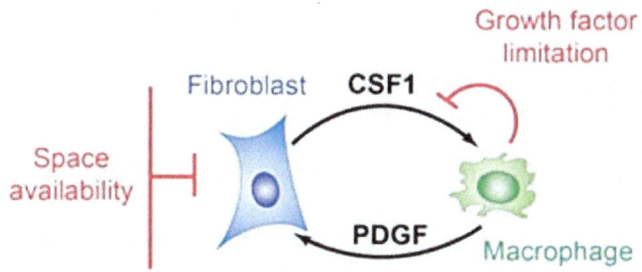

**FIGURE 2-2** Macrophage-fibroblast two-cell circuit.
NOTE: CSF1 = colony stimulating factor 1; PDGF = platelet-derived growth factor.
SOURCES: Medzhitov presentation, November 2, 2021; adapted from Zhou et al., 2018.

he and his colleagues found that the two paradigms are mechanistically coupled, in that space availability for fibroblasts thereby controlled growth factor production for macrophages. Through a homeostatic or density-sensitive enhancer, fibroblasts sense available space and produce the requisite amount of CSF-1 growth factor to generate the number of macrophages that correspond to the available space detected by fibroblasts. In this way, the two paradigms are coupled, he explained.

Macrophage growth factor CSF-1 also has a ubiquitous inflammation-sensitive enhancer that is controlled by nuclear factor kappa B, or NF-kB. This inflammatory enhancer is independent of cellular density and enables macrophages to expand as necessary to support the inflammatory response. This principle of growth factor production—in which one cell type senses the tissue microenvironment and produces growth factor to regulate another cell type—can be further generalized, Medzhitov stated. One well-known example is that oxygen sensed through the hypoxia-inducible factor-1 pathway regulates vascular endothelial growth factor, or VEGF, which in turn controls the appropriate numbers of endothelial cells. The general rule seems to be that one cell type, which senses the microenvironment, is linked to population size control of another cell type, Medzhitov said.

## TISSUE REPAIR AND REGENERATION

Tissues can be described as labile, stable, or permanent based on the type and degree of cell turnover, Medzhitov explained. Labile tissues have stem cells like epithelial cells and hematopoietic cells, and differentiated cells in the tissue are continuously renewed by stem cells. Although labile tissues are easily damaged, they are also easy to repair by way of regeneration, in which lost cells are simply replaced, he said. Stable tissues have some capacity for regeneration if the damage is limited, but if the damage is extensive, repair occurs by fibrosis. In stable tissues, stem-cell–based renewal is not typical; rather, regeneration happens via mitosis of terminally differentiated cells, such as hepatocytes, fibroblasts, and pancreatic beta cells. Comprised of cells like neurons and cardiomyocytes, permanent tissues can only repair by fibrosis, making these tissues vulnerable to degenerative disease. These three classes of tissues have different rules that govern how supportive cells assist functional client cells, how cell population sizes are controlled, and how the tissues repair. He added that the optimal regenerative approach will, therefore, depend on the category to which the target cell belongs.

# 3

# Lessons Learned from Immune Tolerance and Graft Acceptance

---

**Key Points Highlighted by Individual Speakers**

- A microbiome poses a low risk for graft-versus-host disease (GVHD) when it is either healthy and diverse or depleted of bacteria. A microbiome in an unstable state between healthy and depleted poses high risk for GVHD. (Jenq)
- Immunosuppressive drugs have side effects and need to be taken for life; inducing tolerance bypasses many engineering and rejection concerns and leaves the immune system intact. (Sykes)
- Success in regenerative medicine will require advances in (1) development of pluripotent hematopoietic stem cells from human pluripotent stem cells and (2) durable mixed chimerism with nontoxic conditioning. (Sykes)
- New technologies, such as organoid models, could provide a platform for interrogating the parameters of the immune system that affect acceptance or rejection of different cell types and understanding the rules for those interactions. (Medzhitov)
- The approach of reverse translation—from "bench to bedside and back to bench"—can foster hypothesis generation and experimental testing, particularly with a heterogeneous patient population receiving treatments or transplants. (Jenq, Talib)
- Engineering direct differentiation of pluripotent cells to mesenchymal stem cells holds potential for regenerative medicine. (Sykes)

The first session of the workshop explored the current state of knowledge about immune tolerance mechanisms and the lessons learned from other areas of research, including transplant immunology, cancer immunotherapy, and the microbiome. Sohel Talib, scientific program officer at the California Institute for Regenerative Medicine, moderated the session.

## THE MICROBIOME AND IMMUNE TOLERANCE: LESSONS FROM ALLOGENEIC HEMATOPOIETIC CELL TRANSPLANTATION

Robert Jenq, deputy department chair of genomic medicine and associate professor of genomic medicine and stem cell transplantation at the University of Texas MD Anderson Cancer Center, stated that allotransplant is a standard treatment for hematological malignancies and is commonly complicated by graft-versus-host disease (GVHD). Approximately 16 percent of mortality in adults who die within 100 days of unrelated donor hematopoietic cell transplantation (HCT) is attributed to GVHD (Phelan et al., 2020).

### Pathophysiology of Graft-Versus-Host Disease

The paradigm for how GVHD is believed to occur begins with a patient who undergoes chemotherapy, radiation, or immune-depleting antibody treatment to facilitate engraftment of the hematopoietic cell graft from an unrelated donor (Jenq and van den Brink, 2010). The bacterial products within the patient are thought to translocate and activate host antigen–presenting cells, which in turn activate the effector immune system via donor T cells within the stem cell graft, Jenq explained. These donor T cells then recruit other immune pathways through a variety of mechanisms, such as inflammatory cytokines and cytotoxic ligands. The T cells can also recruit other immune cells, including natural killer (NK) cells and macrophages. Together, the T cells and recruited innate myeloid cells can target a variety of tissues. Classically, these targets are the skin, gastrointestinal tract, liver, and hematopoietic system. A "silver lining" of this process, Jenq said, is an antitumor response that occurs during the inflammatory cascade in which the leukemia, lymphoma, or hematological malignancy becomes better controlled.

### *Early Studies and Interventions for Graft-Versus-Host Disease*

The pathophysiology of GVHD is derived from studies conducted over the past century, said Jenq. One of the earliest germ-free isolators was developed in the 1920s. Housing animal subjects, these sterilizable steel isolators featured ports with attached gloves and windows for handling and viewing the subjects. While the isolator design and materials have changed in past decades, the basic features remain the same. In the 1970s, two pioneering papers were published—the first detailed a study conducted on germ-free mice in isolators, and the second looked at normal mice treated with gut-decontaminating antibiotics (Jones et al., 1971; van Bekkum et al., 1974). These two studies indicate that in the absence of a microbiome, GVHD is much milder than it otherwise would be. Thus, the microbiome contributes to the pathophysiology of GVHD, he explained.

The microbiome studies on mice were soon followed by clinical application, Jenq said. In the 1980s, Rainer Storb at the Fred Hutchinson Cancer Center in Seattle studied the effects of sterilization on bone marrow transplant patients. A 1983 study reported findings on patients with severe aplastic anemia who were conditioned with cyclophosphamide, followed by a bone marrow transplant from matched siblings (Storb et al., 1983). Thirty-nine of the 130 patients were randomly assigned to a protective environment with laminar airflow. Food was sterilized, utensils were autoclaved, and any items given to patients were sterilized, encased in plastic, and slipped through a slot in the room. Before examining patients, medical staff took the same precautions normally taken prior to performing surgery. Patients remained in this protective environment for 50 days. The study, Jenq said, suggested a benefit from near-total bacterial decontamination, with a markedly reduced incidence of GVHD in the protective isolation conditions that translated into a sizable improvement in overall survival. Patients in the protective environment had an 87 percent probability of survival, compared to 69 percent for patients in settings without laminar airflow (Storb et al., 1983). Therefore, the protective environment became standard practice in the 1980s and early 1990s. However, later studies did not indicate a clear benefit, and this research—coupled with the expense of providing a protective environment—led to the practice gradually falling out of favor (Passweg et al., 1998; Petersen et al., 1987; Russell et al., 2000). Jenq recalled asking Storb why the results did not hold up; Storb attributed it to the absence of cyclosporine in the earlier study, which was conducted prior to the use of calcineurin inhibitors such as cyclosporine, now commonly used to inhibit T cells and prevent GVHD. Once cyclosporine-based GVHD prophylactic treatment was available, the advantage of protective isolation was no longer as apparent.

### Effect of the Microbiome on Allotransplant Mortality

Two decades later, research continues to focus on whether the microbiome can predict mortality in allotransplant patients, Jenq stated. A multicenter study—with researchers from Memorial Sloan Kettering Cancer Center, Duke University, Regensburg University Hospital, and Hokkaido

University—explored fecal microbiome diversity in transplant patients (Peled et al., 2020). Researchers collected 8,767 fecal samples from 1,362 patients across the globe. Profiling the samples revealed that patients have fairly healthy microbiomes with high diversity when they begin their bone marrow transplant hospitalizations. However, during the course of the two- or three-week hospitalizations, most patients rapidly lose much of that diversity. This finding held across all four research centers and indicates that microbiome diversity matters. Researchers stratified the patients by their microbiome diversity to compare the outcomes of those with higher diversity to those with lower diversity. Patients with higher microbiome diversity had improved overall survival rates compared to their counterparts. Mortality related to GVHD appears to be the primary driver in the difference in overall survival rates, Jenq explained.

Further analysis identified that the use of antibiotics could account for some of the differences in loss of microbiome diversity (Peled et al., 2020). When patients lose neutrophils, they often experience high fevers that are treated with empiric, broad-spectrum antibiotics. However, Jenq said, not all antibiotics are equally harmful to the microbiome. For instance, researchers found that cefepime was not highly associated with loss of diversity, whereas meropenem and piperacillin-tazobactam were more highly associated. Some antibiotic associations were only observed in particular centers, likely due to center-specific practices in first-line treatment for neutropenic fever, Jenq noted.

*Factors Underlying Loss of Microbiome Diversity*

Jenq and his colleagues at MD Anderson Cancer Center have further explored the associations between antibiotics and GVHD. In a study of almost 300 patients with myelodysplastic syndromes or leukemia who received allotransplants, researchers examined the rates of GVHD in patients subgrouped by the antibiotic treatment they received: meropenem, cefepime, both meropenem and cefepime, or no antibiotics. A pattern emerged, with patients that received no antibiotics showing a low incidence of intestinal GVHD (approximately 10 percent). Cefepime, which is not associated with loss of diversity due to its fairly narrow spectrum of activity, showed a similar incidence of GVHD to the group that received no antibiotics. However, patients who received meropenem—either on its own or in combination with cefepime—had a much higher incidence of GVHD, at almost 25 percent.

Retrospective clinical studies may indicate associations, but they do not demonstrate causality, Jenq explained. Therefore, he and his colleagues turned to a mouse model of experimentally induced GVHD (Hayase et al., 2021). Some mice were given transplants with a human leukocyte antigen

(HLA)-identical graft, which avoids GVHD. Other mice received HLA-disparate grafts, leading to the development of GVHD approximately one month post-transplant. Meropenem treatment was added to the drinking water of a third set of mice receiving HLA-disparate grafts, resulting in aggravation of GVHD and providing evidence for causality. Jenq noted that an additional advantage of preclinical animal studies is the opportunity to investigate potential mechanisms. Jenq described the work of Eiko Hayase, postdoctoral fellow at MD Anderson Cancer Center, who explored whether the meropenem was depleting beneficial bacteria or contributing to the expansion of harmful bacteria. Hayase tested for this by adding oral decontamination, and the results were similar to the previously mentioned 1970s decontamination studies in that the mice receiving decontamination and meropenem showed reduced GVHD mortality compared to mice without decontamination. The result indicates that one of the mechanisms of meropenem is selection for a harmful, pro-inflammatory bacterial population, Jenq added.

*Categories of Intestinal Bacteria*

Jenq explained that intestinal bacteria can be either gram positive or negative and are categorized by type of anaerobe, either facultative or obligate. Bacteria that are tolerant of oxygen are facultative anaerobes, and oxygen-intolerant bacteria are obligate anaerobes. Clostridia are gram positive, obligate anaerobes. Generally thought to be friendly commensals, clostridia help digest food, regulate the immune system, and produce short-chain fatty acids that can recruit regulatory T cells and produce nutrients for the epithelium. Another class of bacteria—bacteroidia—are also obligate anaerobes, but they are gram negative. Typically, they are also thought to be friendly commensals, and under normal conditions, bacteroidia help people digest fiber and starches; however, in the absence of fiber and starches, this subpopulation can alter their gene expression and consume mucus as a source of carbohydrates. Jenq explained that Hayase and her colleagues used 16S sequencing to profile the microbiome of mice and compared mice without GVHD, with GVHD, and with GVHD plus meropenem treatment. Clostridia were sensitive to meropenem, shown by loss of bacteria within that class, while *Bacteroides*—a genus within the bacteroidia class—exhibited significant enrichment (Hayase et al., 2021).

*Role of* Bacteroides thetaiotaomicron *in Graft-Versus-Host Disease*

Hayase utilized this information, Jenq said, to add another component to the decontamination model by reintroducing *Bacteroides thetaiotaomicron* (*B. theta*), the predominant bacteroidia species in mice. The introduction of *B. theta* resulted in aggravated GVHD, indicating that *B. theta* is a pro-inflammatory, potentially harmful bacteria, said Jenq. Having broad capability to digest dietary fiber polysaccharides and glycans, *B. theta* is believed to be versatile in its carbohydrate utilization. Cultivating *B. theta* with four different carbohydrates it is capable of consuming has shown that it will not consume all four carbohydrates simultaneously. Instead, *B. theta* will target one carbohydrate until it is depleted, at which point it will target the next carbohydrate. A hierarchy of carbohydrate preference has been found for this organism, Jenq noted. The mice treated with meropenem showed loss of the mucus layer in the colon, leading to increased translocation of bacteria and compromised barrier function. Research on gene expression profiled how *Bacteroides* behave under different conditions (Hayase et al., 2021). Jenq and his colleagues found that (1) the carbohydrate xylose is lost with meropenem treatment and (2) xylose is beneficial for reverting *Bacteroides* back to friendly commensals.

## Applications to Other Fields

Jenq outlined lessons learned from this research that might apply to other fields (see Figure 3-1). When the microbiome is healthy and diverse, it does not contribute to inflammation or to rejection. The removal or depletion of the microbiome—as was done in early studies—also lowers the inflammatory risk. However, a microbiome that is in an unstable state between the two extremes of healthy or depleted poses the largest risk for GVHD, translocation, or alloimmune rejection of stem cells. When asked how an individual at high risk of GVHD can be moved toward a lower-risk microbiome state, Jenq replied that for decades, Leiden University in the Netherlands has used an approach to avoid the high-risk microbiome state. It involves decontamination until the greatest risk for GVHD has passed. Once the patient's neutrophils have recovered and cytokine levels

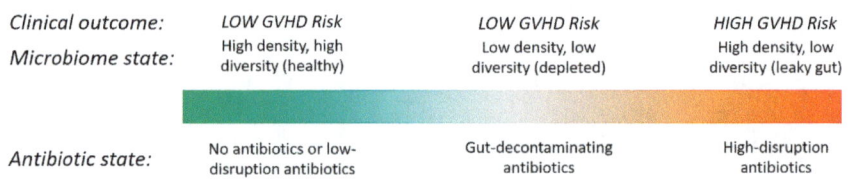

**FIGURE 3-1** Microbiome and antibiotic states and clinical risk of graft-versus-host disease.
NOTE: GVHD = graft-versus-host disease.
SOURCES: Adapted from Jenq presentation, November 2, 2021; Schwabkey and Jenq, 2020.

have settled, microbiome diversity and colonization resistance are rapidly restored through a fecal transplant.

## IMMUNE TOLERANCE AND GRAFT ACCEPTANCE: LESSONS FROM TRANSPLANT IMMUNOLOGY

Megan Sykes, Michael J. Friedlander Professor of Medicine, professor of microbiology and immunology and surgical sciences (in surgery) and director of the Columbia Center for Translational Immunology at Columbia University, provided an overview of lessons learned from transplant immunology with application to immune tolerance and graft acceptance. The success of organ transplantation depends on immunosuppressant drugs that must be taken for life and are broadly immunosuppressive, Sykes said. Complications associated with immunosuppression include viral reactivation, susceptibility to cancer, and side effects such as diabetes and kidney toxicity, among others. These drug treatment–related complications are a major limitation to the success of organ transplantation. Furthermore, late graft rejection due to a chronic immune response is an ongoing problem. The holy grail in the field of organ transplantation, Sykes said, is to induce immune tolerance, thus avoiding the need for immunosuppressive drugs. Immune tolerance can be defined as "long-term graft acceptance with normal immunocompetence without requiring immunosuppressive therapy," she said. Tolerance retains normal immune function, preserving the ability to resist infection and cancer.

### Cell Engineering to Avoid Graft Rejection

An alternative strategy to tolerance, Sykes highlighted, is cell engineering to avoid the rejection of tissues, and possibly organs, derived from pluripotent hematopoietic stem cells. Current research is exploring the removal of major histocompatibility complex (MHC) molecules—the HLA—from such stem cells to avoid recognition by T lymphocytes, which are the major drivers of immune rejection. Although the removal of HLA enables cells to evade T-cell immunity, the cells are more susceptible to NK cell–mediated rejection. Evading T-cell immunity would also result in the loss of normal tumor surveillance on the transplanted cells and the inability to protect the graft from infections. Sykes noted that other approaches, such as expressing immunosuppressive molecules like programmed death-ligand 1 (PD-L1), do not involve HLA removal. However, concerns about the susceptibility of organs or tissues to infection persist with these approaches. Immune tolerance is not associated with these concerns, Sykes said, and is therefore a viable alternative approach to achieve acceptance of pluripotent stem-cell–derived grafts.

*Mechanisms of Immune Tolerance and Allograft Tolerance Induction*

There are three major mechanisms of tolerance: clonal deletion, anergy, and suppression. In clonal deletion, the cells that recognize the donor antigens, such as T cells, are not present, Sykes explained. With anergy, T cells persist but no longer respond to the antigen through their T-cell receptors. In suppression, T cells persist but are actively suppressed, for example, through regulatory T cells (Tregs). Allograft tolerance induction has been explored in the transplantation field for many years, resulting in thousands of reports of successful tolerance induction, said Sykes, though most of these results involved rodents and vascularized allografts, which are highly tolerogenic. A T-cell response involves both a destructive response and a suppressive, regulatory response, and it appears that rodent vascularized allografts have a strong ability to induce suppressive Treg responses. Partial or temporary immunosuppression allows this regulatory response to dominate, leading to graft acceptance. However, these approaches have rarely been successfully applied in large animal models and humans, Sykes added.

### Regulatory Cell Therapies in Clinical Trials of Organ Transplantation

Several regulatory cell therapies are currently being explored in clinical trials. One approach involves cell therapy of various cell types that have demonstrated a regulatory function in animal models, said Sykes. Multiple clinical trials in HCT and organ transplantation are examining Tregs. These trials include three types of Tregs: (1) polyclonal cells that are nonspecifically expanded ex vivo, (2) cells that are expanded ex vivo in response to donor antigens, and (3) cells into which a chimeric antigen receptor has been introduced. Other studies explore approaches that involve regulatory dendritic cells, mesenchymal stem cells, and tolerogenic monocytes. None of the trials of these various approaches have an endpoint of complete immunosuppression withdrawal, Sykes said; therefore, they do not assess allograft tolerance. The only way to test tolerance would be to completely remove immunosuppression, which denies the patient the standard of care. This approach would not be attempted unless allograft tolerance were achieved in large animal models, and thus far these approaches generally have not been shown to achieve tolerance.

Efficacy data in the most stringent rodent models—such as skin grafts mismatched for MHC—as well as efficacy and safety data in large animal preclinical models might be needed before clinical trials in tolerance induction and immunosuppression removal should begin, Sykes suggested. A good model of transplant rejection of all kinds has been established in nonhuman primates, she noted. Furthermore, safety data for the proposed drugs or biological agents in humans are required. HCT has been explored in large animal models and is the approach that comes the closest to meeting these criteria, and it has been tested in immunosuppression withdrawal trials in humans, Sykes added.

*Non-Myeloablative Mixed Chimerism Protocol Studies*

Hematopoietic stem cell transplantation (HSCT) can cause GVHD and other toxic side effects, and thus cannot be used in its traditional form in a person who needs an organ transplant but who does not have a hematological malignancy, Sykes explained. Meeting the requirements of HCT for tolerance induction is a challenge in the field; it involves developing a minimally toxic, non-myeloablative conditioning regimen that allows hematopoietic cell engraftments across HLA barriers while completely avoiding GVHD. This has been achieved in mice through non-myeloablative mixed chimerism protocols. An early model specifically targeted recipient T cells in the periphery with monoclonal antibodies and in the thymus with local irradiation to the thymus, combined with a low dose of total body irradiation (Sharabi and Sachs, 1989). This model achieved mixed hematopoietic chimerism in which donor and host cells coexisted for life, and the recipient animals were tolerant to the donor.

*Pure Deletional Tolerance through Durable Mixed Chimerism*

Mechanisms of this and other regimens have since been shown to involve depletion of alloreactive T cells in both the peripheral and thymic compartments, said Sykes. Donor hematopoietic stem cells are grafted in the bone marrow, and these hematopoietic stem cells then send progeny and coexisting recipient cells to the recipient thymus. This leads to the production of dendritic cells that mediate clonal deletion of newly developing T cells, allowing the tolerant T cells to fill the depleted peripheral T-cell compartment. The emerging T cells are tolerant of the donor and recipient, creating a centrally tolerized T-cell compartment. The procedure ultimately yields lifelong mixed chimerism and donor-specific tolerance, Sykes explained.

Although achieving this process in large animals and humans has been elusive thus far, Sykes said, other animal models, primarily rodents, have shown the complete deletion of donor-reactive cells. Pure deletional tolerance, with no long-term role for regulatory mechanisms, has been observed when durable mixed chimerism is achieved with complete, global T-cell ablation in the periphery and thymus (Khan et al., 1996; Nikolic et al., 2001; Sharabi et al., 1990; Tomita et al., 1994). It has also been accomplished with other models that specifically remove preexisting donor-reactive T cells in the periphery and thymus—without global depletion—by combining costimulatory blockade with the bone marrow transplant (Fehr et al., 2008; Fehr et al., 2010; Fehr et al., 2005; Haspot et al., 2008; Kurtz et al., 2004; Lucas et al., 2011; Takeuchi et al., 2004). In other models, complete deletion of donor-reactive cells was not achieved; instead, Tregs were expanded in response to the donor, resulting in a combination of Treg mediation and ongoing central deletional tolerance (Bemelman et al., 1998; Bigenzahn et al., 2005; Domenig et al., 2005; Yamazaki et al., 2007). The combination of regulation and deletion can be a powerful method for inducing tolerance, Sykes emphasized.

### Hematopoietic Stem Cell Transplantation for Kidney Allograft Tolerance

Three clinical trials of HSCT for kidney allograft tolerance have been conducted. While working at Massachusetts General Hospital (MGH), Sykes and her colleagues carried out a study involving non-myeloablative conditioning and succeeded in achieving tolerance across HLA barriers, which she noted is the most challenging immunological barrier. Northwestern University also achieved tolerance in HLA-mismatched full chimeras; however, the regimen was associated with GVHD and infectious complications. This trial is now in phase III. Stanford University tested another regimen that achieved mixed chimerism, but has thus far only worked in HLA-identical transplants and has not yet been successfully achieved in HLA-mismatched trials. Samsung Medical Center in South Korea is currently testing a protocol similar to that of MGH.

### Translational Studies between Hematopoietic Cell Transplantation and Organ Transplantation

Translational work between HCT and organ transplantation led to the MGH protocol, Sykes said. While testing a monkey model, she and her colleagues learned that transient mixed chimerism associated with HCT transplantation at the time of kidney transplant from the same donor could lead to tolerance. This discovery led to successful tolerance protocols supported by the Immune Tolerance Network (Kawai et al., 2008; Kawai et al., 2013). The chimerism lasted only a few weeks, and therefore the long-term central deletional mechanism of tolerance referenced earlier could not be applied to these patients (LoCascio et al., 2010). Sykes and her colleagues studied the mechanisms of tolerance in these patients and developed a method of identifying the alloreactive repertoire based on T-cell receptor sequencing (Morris et al., 2015). In tracking these data, researchers found deletion of preexisting donor-reactive T cells in long-term patients (Morris et al., 2015). Furthermore, a specific expansion of donor-specific Treg clones was observed during the early period (Savage et al., 2018). This transient chimerism leverages two mechanisms of tolerance, combining the early role of expanded donor-specific Tregs with the long-term deletion of preexisting donor-reactive T cells, Sykes explained.

*Overcoming Limitations of Transient Chimerism*

While this approach has worked in monkey models of kidney transplantation, it has not worked for other organs that are not tolerogenic, such as lung, liver, heart, or islets of Langerhans in the pancreas. Sykes outlined several limitations of transient chimerism: (1) the kidney plays an important role in promoting tolerance and must be grafted with the bone marrow transplant, (2) not all organs are tolerogenic like the kidney, and (3) no success has yet been achieved with a regimen that would be relevant for cadaveric donation. To help overcome these limitations, she and her colleagues at Columbia University have established a nonhuman primate transplant program aimed at creating a more durable mixed chimerism that will succeed for all types of organs. They use a non-myeloablative model that builds on previous transient chimerism studies and adds autologous polyclonal Tregs. The kidney graft is delayed to four months after the bone marrow transplant in order to conduct a stringent test of bone marrow–induced tolerance. The kidney is known to promote tolerance, she noted, and therefore if tolerance persists to 120 days without the kidney graft, then the model does not rely on the kidney itself for tolerance induction. They found that when a donor kidney was transplanted into the animal four months after the bone marrow transplant, the kidney was accepted with no immunosuppression and showed no infiltrates (Duran-Struuck et al., 2017). The control group did not receive Tregs, and these animals rejected the delayed kidney transplants. The results demonstrate that the combination of Tregs and a low-intensity conditioning regimen can achieve more robust tolerance than has previously been seen, Sykes explained. This tolerance does not depend upon the presence of the donor kidney, and therefore it should be applicable to other types of transplants.

## Applications of Immune Tolerance and Graft Acceptance to Regenerative Medicine

Sykes outlined the relevance of immune tolerance and graft acceptance to regenerative medicine. The transplant community is working to develop gentler, non-myeloablative regimens for mixed chimerism induction that foster systemic tolerance to the donor. Several groups are advancing the development of pluripotent hematopoietic stem cells from human pluripotent stem cells. Advances will continue in the achievement of durable mixed chimerism with relatively nontoxic conditioning regimens, she said.

Success in these two areas could result in an off-the-shelf, pluripotent stem cell-derived donor HSCT that could be used to achieve tolerance for organs and tissues derived from those same pluripotent stem cells. This approach is optimal because it does not require the graft to be immunosuppressive; rather, the entire recipient immune system remains functional and becomes donor-tolerant, Sykes remarked.

## DISCUSSION

### Microbiome Manipulation

Immune system cells play a role in the suppression of GVHD, said Talib, and those cells have their own metabolism that influences GVHD suppression. He asked whether genetic engineering can be used to manipulate the microbiome to aid in engraftment, allograft acceptance, or the suppression of GVHD. Jenq replied that the microbiome was traditionally believed to be limited to epithelial surfaces such as the gastrointestinal tract, the skin, and perhaps the genital urinary tract. However, studies indicate the possibility of a circulating microbiome that can be detected in the blood. Research is also exploring a tumor microbiome, with studies examining viable bacteria within tumor cells in the context of pancreatic and colon cancer. Thus, the belief that the microbiome is only on epithelial surfaces is shifting, he added. Engineering the microbiome is an area of active study, as groups work toward genetic manipulation of bacteria. The tools to genetically manipulate commensal bacteria are limited, and each tool developed only works for a particular species or closely related strains of bacteria. *Lactobacilli*, *Escherichia coli*, and *Bacteroides* are easy to genetically manipulate, while clostridia are substantially more challenging, said Jenq. Therefore, the target for genetic manipulation should be carefully considered. Once the modality is developed, a researcher can be creative in terms of the bacteria that can potentially be made, he added.

### Effects of Systemic Homeostasis and Inflammation on Immune Response

Given that most work on immune response and regeneration focuses on the local niche yet is also influenced by systemic immune homeostasis, Talib asked how systems-level immune function dysregulation can be understood and manipulated to aid local regeneration. Ruslan Medzhitov, Sterling Professor of Immunobiology at Yale University School of Medicine, replied that most knowledge about the effects of systemic homeostasis on local immune function is in regard to systemic metabolic homeostasis—that is, the availability of different types of metabolic fuels such as glucose, fatty acids, and ketones. Other aspects of systemic homeostasis are less clearly understood. Systemic control of core body temperature has long generated interest because it changes with fever during infection, but the influence of increased body temperature on immune function remains unclear after many years of research. Some systemic homeostatic circuits, such as calcium concentration, are so tightly controlled that little variation is allowed. Generally, systemic homeostasis creates indirect effects as it translates to tissue-level homeostasis. Aside from metabolic homeostasis, these effects and the quantitative degree to which they are meaningful are not yet known, said Medzhitov.

Talib asked whether the role of inflammation in immune response could be reappropriated, and if so, what threshold of inflammation would be necessary to initiate a protective immune response. Traditionally, inflammation was viewed as a response to tissue injury or infection, Medzhitov said, whereas current thinking places that type of inflammatory response at one end of a spectrum. Homeostasis is at the other end of the spectrum, and between the endpoints are deviations from homeostasis that are less extreme than the inflammatory response to injury or infection. The question of how much inflammation is necessary to initiate the immune response is complex, because not all immune responses are the same, he said. Measuring a quantitative aspect—such as the amount of cytokines produced—will not fully capture the immune response. Generally, immune responses have been primarily considered from the perspective of defense from microbes, he added. This perspective is shifting as the idea that immune responses might have other functions unrelated to antimicrobial defense garners more attention. The role of inflammation for such immune responses likely differs from that for responses associated with antimicrobial need. This area of research is emerging, as most knowledge of the immune system is based on antimicrobial functions, Medzhitov commented.

## Mechanisms of Tolerance in HLA-mismatched Transplants

Given that the MGH protocol can generate tolerance in HLA-identical or mismatched transplants, whereas the protocol from Stanford University has only been able to generate tolerance in HLA-matched transplants, Talib asked how these protocols differ and what lessons from the differences can be applied to tolerance induction in HLA-mismatched cases. Overall, the two protocols are quite different, Sykes said. The MGH protocol involves pre-transplant non-myeloablative doses of cyclophosphamide, a monoclonal antibody against cluster of differentiation 2 (CD2) to exhaustively deplete peripheral T cells, thymic irradiation to deplete existing alloreactive thymocytes, and a short course of calcineurin inhibitor post-transplant.

The Stanford protocol is based on total lymphoid irradiation and antithymocyte globulin, followed by an association with the kidney transplant, and then a delayed donor HCT.

Sykes noted that Dixon Kaufman, of University of Wisconsin Health, is currently evaluating the Stanford protocol in a nonhuman primate model in an effort to achieve tolerance across MHC barriers. Mechanistic studies are needed to explain how the tolerance is achieved and why it fails when HLA barriers are crossed. The Kaufman study has found that when immunosuppression—in the form of two post-transplant drugs—is stopped, the chimerism disappears and rejection occurs. In the MGH protocol, the chimerism is more transient, yet the graft is not rejected despite the loss of chimerism, she explained. Research on the mechanisms involved indicates expansion of donor-specific Tregs in the early period. This may partly depend on the way in which anti-CD2 selectively spares Tregs while depleting effector memory cells. Each method entails a different combination of mechanisms involving regulation and, to some extent, deletion. Modeling these protocols in nonhuman primates first allows researchers to better understand what to expect for results in humans, she said.

### Tolerance Induction in Xenotransplantation

Given the advancement of genetic engineering, a participant asked Sykes about her thoughts on xenotransplantation. Sykes and her colleagues are currently exploring tolerance induction to xenografts. Immune responses against xenografts are more formidable and involve more mechanisms than responses to allografts, she said. In the allograft response, for instance, when the T-cell response in the naïve recipient is targeted, the response can be overcome, and no other significant activity takes place. In xenotransplantation, natural antibodies independent of T cells, in addition to NK cells, increase innate recognition of the xenograft, creating a much more powerful indirect T-cell response. Thus, the xenograft barrier is stronger, and studying xenograft tolerance is therefore important, Sykes said.

Genetic engineering is a key aspect of preventing xenograft rejection by natural antibodies, which has already been demonstrated with the development of Galalpha1-3Galbeta1-4GlcNAc (Gal) knockout pigs, she added. The combination of genetic engineering and tolerance mechanisms will likely lead to advances. Sykes and her team are specifically targeting their genetic engineering approach to make the bone marrow of pigs better able to survive in a human marrow microenvironment and to resist immediate rejection by human macrophages. Although genetic engineering is a useful tool that helped researchers move past hyperacute rejection, removing additional natural antibody carbohydrate targets of the xenograft, beyond that accomplished with Gal, will not necessarily be the best solution to non-Gal natural antibody-mediated rejection, said Sykes. Further study in nonhuman primates could help make that determination. Some data suggest that removing too many carbohydrate terminal sugars can reveal other natural antibody targets. For this reason, Sykes prefers the mixed chimerism approach because it tolerizes both the T cells and the natural antibody-producing B cells. She and her colleagues are working toward a goal of establishing permanent mixed chimerism in the nonhuman primate model.

### Regulatory T-Cell Expansion

Belumosudil, which inhibits ROCK2,[1] has been approved by the U.S. Food and Drug Administration for chronic GVHD, Talib noted. Given that ROCK2 regulates T helper 17 cells (Th17), he asked whether a ROCK2 inhibitor might increase endogenous Tregs and be used in place of anti-thymocyte globulin to help suppress GVHD for solid organ transplants. Sykes replied that Treg instability is a major limitation in the use of exogenous Tregs and has been a barrier in extending studies to additional animals. The inflammatory environment produced by conditioning and lymphopenia contains substantial interleukin 6 (IL6). Current understanding is that Tregs in that environment may deviate toward the Th17 phenotype. Determining how to control this tendency is a challenge for researchers. Expanding endogenous Tregs is a research area of interest, Sykes noted. Approaches to supporting the survival and stability of infused Tregs are being explored, and clinical trials are conducting safety tests on methods to expand endogenous Tregs via drugs or cytokines and on several cell-based mechanisms. Tolerogenic dendritic cells and mesenchymal stem cells have been shown to be associated with expanded donor-specific Tregs. Engineering the population of antigen-presenting cells is one approach that will likely be an important component of a robust tolerance regimen, Sykes said.

### Blocking the Initiation of Immune Response

A participant asked how the immune system's potential can be harnessed to improve patient responses to regenerative therapies. Opportunities for transplantation depend on the type of tissue involved, Medzhitov said, as well as the cell type and its role within the tissue. Transplanted cells require appropriate growth factors in the extracellular matrix in order to survive, flourish, and differentiate. They also need to be protected from

---

[1] ROCK2 is the abbreviated name for rho-associated coiled-coil-containing protein kinase. It is involved in a signaling pathway that regulates the balance between regulatory T cells and T helper 17 cells (Jagasia et al., 2021).

destructive aspects of the immune response. Two strategies for protecting the transplanted cells include (1) suppressing the response, which involves unwanted side effects, or (2) blocking signals that initiate the immune response. This second strategy could lead to a more desirable outcome because the immune system is not suppressed indiscriminately and remains functional, yet it is prevented from attacking transplanted cells. Achieving this outcome will require understanding the signals involved in recognition beyond matching molecular signatures. The immune system may be put on alert both because of a foreign signal from a mismatched MHC or microbial foreign antigen and because of a loss of normal homeostasis within the tissue. These functions of the immune system are noncanonical since they do not involve antimicrobial defense. Better understanding of such immune system inputs is necessary to pursue the preferred strategy of preventing activation of the immune system rather than suppressing an ongoing immune response, he said.

## Organoid Models

Given that tissues have specific immune environments with tissue-resident immune cells playing an important role, Talib asked how organoid models with induced pluripotent stem cells can be used to understand the local immune system environment and improve methods for tissue and cell transplantation. Medzhitov replied that these technologies are proving to be incredibly powerful, but their full power will be realized when organoids incorporate more cell types and when they become self-sufficient such that they no longer require exogenous provision of growth factors. This development could provide a platform for interrogating all the parameters of the system that affect acceptance or rejection of different cell types, which could lead to an understanding of the rules that govern those interactions. Personalizing organoid models allows analysis of the role of particular genetic variance on organ function and immune susceptibility, Sykes added. This type of analysis has benefited the ability to generate insulin-producing beta cells from stem cells, she noted. Various types of organoids and chromatin immunoprecipitation assays can be used in high-throughput screening, Jenq said. Since organoid systems can directly study human cells, they circumvent concerns about whether findings in animal studies will hold up in human biology. Although there are challenges associated, some researchers have begun introducing bacteria or a combination of epithelial cells, immune cells, and bacteria to organoid systems, Jenq noted.

## Applying Lessons from COVID-19 to Regenerative Medicine

The COVID-19 pandemic has increased the pace of science, Talib said. He asked whether any lessons from COVID-19 could be applied to move the field of regenerative medicine forward. Sykes remarked that although transplant patients are susceptible to COVID-19, the disease has not been particularly worse for them than for other patient groups. She added, it is not clear that immunosuppression increases the severity of COVID-19 and researchers need to learn more about the pathogenesis of the virus and how the timing and context of the immune system's components affect its role in combating COVID-19. Furthermore, transplant patients and other people with compromised immune systems have not had optimal responses to COVID-19 vaccination, said Sykes. Messenger RNA (mRNA) vaccines have potential applications beyond infectious disease, and researchers are exploring their use in tolerance induction. Enabled by an infusion of funding, the development of COVID-19 vaccines is an "incredible tour de force" that demonstrates how increases in collaboration and energy dedicated to an issue can result in great strides made in a shorter time period, she said. Since the simple, underlying method of manipulating biological systems can be a tool for study to encode anything of interest, mRNA vaccines likely have uses beyond disease treatment and immunity, Medzhitov said. He noted that the COVID-19 pandemic has demonstrated the critical nature of reducing the time from discovery to dissemination of information. The current lengthy process in making research findings broadly available to scientists and the public is unsustainable and should be addressed, Medzhitov remarked.

## Applying Lessons from Transplantation Immunology to Regenerative Medicine

Talib asked the panelists for their final thoughts on how lessons learned from transplantation immunology can be applied to regenerative medicine. History indicates that the most impressive advances in science are not spurred by funding, but by a research area that attracts interest in exploration, Medzhitov stated. Development of technology and tools can increase the feasibility of answering interesting questions. He remarked that making regenerative medicine more attractive through tool development could be a tipping point for the field, given that interesting questions beyond practical implications are already being asked. Sykes emphasized the potential benefits of engineering or directly differentiating pluripotent stem cells into hematopoietic stem cells. Greater investment in this effort could increase progress to benefit tolerance induction and the field of regenerative medicine as a whole. Jenq advocated for the approach of reverse translation, involving a heterogeneous patient population. The approach is fertile ground for generating hypotheses and experimental testing, he continued. Talib added that the California Institute of Regenerative Medicine utilizes this type of approach in "translation going from bench to bedside and from bedside back to the bench" to better understand basic biology or immunology to advance the field.

# 4

# Engineering of Allogeneic Donor Cells for Acceptance by the Host's Immune System

**Key Points Highlighted by Individual Speakers**

- Protecting allogeneic cells from immune destruction is key to unlocking the potential of regenerative medicine. Cellular transplantation without immunosuppression appears to be an achievable goal through the use of hypoimmune cells. (Schrepfer)
- Hypoimmune cells evade allogeneic immune rejection, do not activate a response from natural killer cells and macrophages, can be transplanted into sensitized patients, and do not alter the recipient's immune system. (Schrepfer)
- Markers of disease activity and predictors of mesenchymal stromal cell (MSC) effect should be incorporated into patient selection to optimize the identification of patients who will respond well to MSC treatment. (Le Blanc)
- Fate Therapeutics is focused on producing multiple off-the-shelf chimeric antigen receptor T-cell therapies. (Valamehr)
- Fate Therapeutics uses three strategies to evade the immune system: cloaking to block detection, elimination by monoclonal antibody to deplete the activated immune cell compartment, and attack and proliferation in which a synthetic receptor eliminates reactive cells and promotes positive cellular proliferation. (Valamehr)
- Key strategies for developing successful therapies via target profiles for the cellular product and optimal patient responders:

- Clinical diagnoses should incorporate biological markers in addition to symptoms. (Le Blanc)
- Immune evasion avoids the need for a perfect patient profile. (Schrepfer)
- The cellular therapy approach should be universal and target both the disease (cancer) and the immune system in multiple ways. (Valamehr)
- The vision for the future of cellular therapies is "immunosuppression free." (Schrepfer)

The objective of the second session of the workshop was to explore recent advances in engineering allogeneic donor cells for acceptance by a host's immune system, including gene editing approaches, universal donor cells, and immune evasion. Rachel Salzman, of the American Society of Gene and Cell Therapy, moderated the session.

## MESENCHYMAL STROMAL CELLS IN IMMUNOMODULATORY THERAPIES

Katarina Le Blanc, professor of clinical stem cell research at the Karolinska Institute, discussed efforts to bring mesenchymal stromal cells (MSC) into the clinic with immunomodulatory therapies.

### Function of Mesenchymal Stromal Cells in Multimodal Immunomodulation

Le Blanc provided an overview of the role of mesenchymal stromal cells in multimodal immunomodulation. MSCs interact in a number of ways with both innate and adaptive immune cells, with the end result being induction of regulatory T cells (Treg), she explained (Le Blanc and Mougiakakos, 2012). The mode of action of MSCs applied as a local injection is likely less complex than that of MSCs administered by intravenous infusion (Krampera and Le Blanc, 2021). This may explain why the majority of applications approved by regulatory agencies are delivered locally, she noted. Endothelial cells that are normally in contact with blood have anticoagulant properties, but when an injury ruptures the endothelial layers, MSCs, which are tissue-resident cells, can come into contact with blood. MSCs express surface markers that trigger platelet aggregation and coagulation cascade activation (Moll et al., 2014; Moll et al., 2011; Moll et al., 2012). In addition, MSCs activate the complement system, facilitating MSC engulfment by phagocytes (Gavin et al., 2019b). This reaction is termed the instant blood-mediated inflammatory reaction, and it results in intravenously infused MSCs clotting in the lungs (de Witte et al., 2017; Goncalves et al., 2017). Cytotoxic cells further activate lysosomes and phagocytes that engulf membrane particles and secrete anti-inflammatory factors.

### Mesenchymal Stromal Cell Therapies

The anti-inflammatory properties of MSCs through intravenous infusion and local injection have been evaluated in clinical trials for a number of diseases, Le Blanc said.[1] Although clinical experience confirms an exceptional safety profile, the efficacy of MSC therapy has been difficult to establish. This may be due in part to the tendency to generalize and combine results from different types of MSCs and patients with diverse disease characteristics. Although MSCs from different tissues may look similar under the microscope, they differ greatly in terms of functional characteristics. For instance, research has demonstrated that MSCs from one individual's adipose tissue more closely resemble MSCs from another person's adipose tissue than MSCs from the individual's own bone marrow (Gregoire et al., 2019; Ho et al., 2018; Kehl et al., 2019; Menard et al., 2020; Menard et al., 2013). This result indicates tissue specificity in MSCs, Le Blanc emphasized. Furthermore, the pro-coagulant properties differ depending on the tissue of origin (Moll et al., 2014; Moll et al., 2012). For example, MSCs derived from placenta induced massive clotting in comparison to MSCs from bone marrow. The coagulation activation of MSCs from the umbilical cord and adipose tissue falls in between that of MSCs from placenta and bone marrow. Finally, primary fibroblasts induced massive clotting (Moll et al., 2014; Moll et al., 2012), she noted.

#### Role of the Recipient in Mesenchymal Stromal Cell Treatments

Projecting the effect of MSC treatment requires an understanding of the recipients, Le Blanc remarked. Most diseases are classified based on clinical features, without full understanding of the underlying disease biology, she added. For instance, Le Blanc and her colleagues examined the gut mucosa of patients who fulfilled clinical criteria for severe GVHD (Gavin et al., 2019a). Biopsies of gut mucosa were obtained prior to the MSC infusion, and gross histological staining and immunohistochemistry were

---

[1] Intravenous infusion: graft-versus-host disease; multiple sclerosis; solid organ transplantation; myocardial infarction; heart failure; Crohn's disease fistulas; asthma; aging frailty; acute respiratory distress syndrome. Local injection: vocal fold scarring; xerostomia; radiation injury; Beurger's disease; osteoarthritis.

used to assess the immune cell profiles. From a biological point of view, samples from the patients who responded to MSC treatment differed in appearance from those of nonresponders, Le Blanc explained. In line with these findings, another study found that GVHD patients with high cytotoxic activity against the infused MSCs during in vitro testing were more likely to respond to MSC therapy (Galleu et al., 2017). Both studies found differences in the cells of responders compared to those of nonresponders, Le Blanc highlighted.

Another study found that patients with high levels of established markers of poor prognosis were more likely to benefit from MSC infusion, Le Blanc noted (Kasikis et al., 2021). Patients with poor prognosis were given the MSC treatment remestemcel-L or the best available therapy. The risk of death six months post-transplant was compared for both groups of patients, and those who received MSC treatment in the high-risk group were more likely to survive, she said. In a trial for chronic GVHD, an immunological analysis indicated that patients who responded to MSC therapy had higher levels of naïve T and B cells than nonresponder patients did. Unlike their counterparts, responder patients mobilized Tregs rapidly after each infusion (Boberg et al., 2020). Within hours or days after each infusion, specific cytokine responses to infused MSCs were evident in responder patients and were maintained for subsequent treatments. The results suggest that there are clear differences between those who respond to MSC treatment and those who do not, Le Blanc remarked.

*Potential Markers of Responsiveness to Mesenchymal Stromal Cell Therapies*

Le Blanc commented that she and Mauro Krampera, a collaborator of hers from the University of Verona, were asked to speculate on the markers that could predict responsiveness to MSCs or indicate patient responses after infusions. They separated biomarkers of disease activity from markers of MSC effect (Krampera and Le Blanc, 2021). Understanding the biological markers of disease activity may be crucial in future patient selection efforts, she noted. A diagnosis made solely on clinical symptoms will never allow optimal patient selection, she reiterated. The algorithms involved are quite complex, and much remains to be learned about MSC clinical use. This may be another reason why the MSC products approved to-date largely employ local injection. Accumulating clinical data will aid in selecting patients most likely to benefit from MSC treatment, she added.

## PROTECTING TRANSPLANTED CELLS FROM IMMUNE REJECTION

Sonja Schrepfer, head of the hypoimmune platform at Sana Biotechnology and professor of surgery at University of California, San Francisco, described approaches to protecting transplanted cells from immune rejection, which she called "one of the keys to unlock the potential for the regenerative medicine field."

### Regenerative Stem Cell Therapy

Even recent advances in stem cell biology can be associated with immune recognition and rejection. One might assume that a stem cell therapy approach that regenerates a patient's own cells and transplants them back into that same patient would avoid immune recognition or rejection of the graft, said Schrepfer (see Figure 4-1). However, the immune system can recognize autologous cell products that are generated from the same patient's cells (Deuse et al., 2019; Deuse et al., 2015). Another approach produces induced pluripotent stem cells (iPSCs) from a group of healthy human leukocyte antigen (HLA) donors with different HLA types (Kawamura et al., 2016). The iPSCs are then banked in off-the-shelf formulas to use in allogeneic transplantation into HLA-matched patients. This approach is based on the theory that HLA molecules serve as a fingerprint of the cell that is recognized as foreign when transplanting cells from one person to another and that rejection will not take place when the fingerprints match, she said. Both approaches have resulted in cases of antigen recognition of the alloantigen, Schrepfer noted. In addition to the contribution of HLA in immune recognition and rejection, molecules such as minor histocompatibility antigens (miHA) can also be recognized. Autologous cell products carry the risk that miHA neoantigens will form and allogeneic HLA-matched cell products from HLA banks can also present miHA, leading to immune rejection.

### Autologous Regenerative Stem Cell Therapy

In the autologous cell products approach, somatic cells from a patient hospitalized with organ failure, for example, are isolated and reprogrammed into iPSCs, Schrepfer explained. This reprogramming generates an autologous cell product that is then transplanted back into the same patient. Because the cells are harvested from the patient who will receive the cell product, it is expected that mismatch will be avoided and that the immune system will recognize the transplant as autologous and not become activated. However, this does not always prove to be the case. For example,

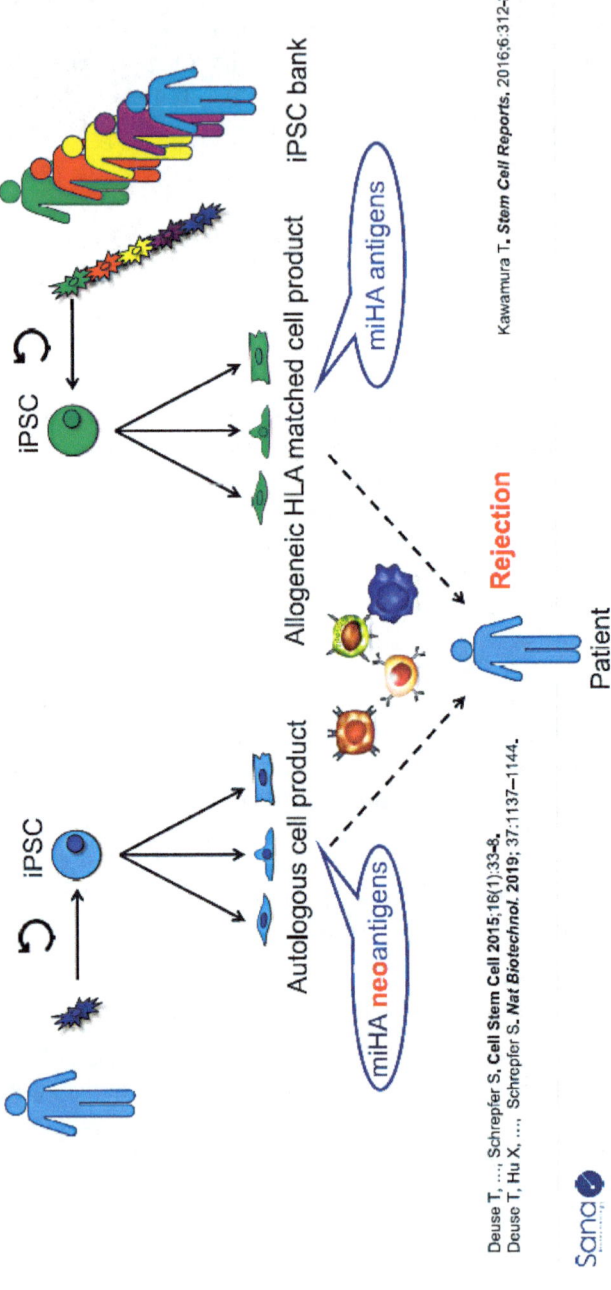

**FIGURE 4-1** Overview of regenerative stem cell therapy.
NOTE: HLA = human leukocyte antigen; iPSC = induced pluripotent stem cells; miHA = minor histocompatibility antigens.
SOURCE: Schrepfer presentation, November 2, 2021.

a cell type such as a cardiomyocyte has mitochondria that carry mitochondrial DNA (mtDNA), which is not as well protected as nuclear DNA, meaning that mtDNA mutations can occur, said Schrepfer. The mtDNA codes for 13 proteins within the respiratory chain; any mutations to these proteins will cause the immune system to recognize the cells as foreign, which could trigger immunoactivation (Deuse et al., 2019).

Fibroblasts from six mice were isolated, reprogrammed into iPSCs, and then cultured in a study that illustrated some of the immunological hurdles related to autologous cell products in regenerative stem cell therapy (Deuse et al., 2019; Deuse et al., 2015). Over time, the iPSCs were passaged, or split, numerous times, Schrepfer described. Researchers found that iPSCs that were passaged 37 (P37) times had a higher frequency of mutations in mtDNA than did iPSCs passaged 7 (P7) times. In a heat map of mtDNA sequencing data, P37 mitochondrially encoded cytochrome c oxidase I—also called Co1—was found to have 92 percent heteroplasmy, meaning that 92 percent of the mitochondria in the cells carried that mutation. After transplanting these cells into the same mouse they were originally harvested from—an autologous or syngeneic transplant setting—researchers found that all the P7 cells survived. In contrast, when P37 cells were transplanted, only 40 percent of the grafted cells survived and the grafts in three of the mice were rejected. This indicates that the immune system can recognize even a single nucleotide polymorphism, demonstrating that autologous HLA can present neoantigens leading to rejection of autologous iPSCs, Schrepfer explained.

## Human Leukocyte Antigen Banking for Pluripotent Stem Cells

The HLA banking concept aims to achieve matched transplantation that avoids autoimmune recognition, which has been tested by Teruhisa Kawamura and colleagues, said Schrepfer (Kawamura et al., 2016). Nonhuman primates (NHPs) matched for major histocompatibility complex (MHC) were used to imitate an HLA bank for humans. Researchers transplanted iPSC-generated cardiomyocyte patches under the skin of recipient MHC-matched monkeys and then grouped them by immunosuppression treatment administration. One group received no immunosuppression, and despite using MHC-matched grafts, all grafts in this group were rejected. Another group received tacrolimus with trough levels above 10 nanograms per milliliter, which is equivalent to what would be administered to a transplant patient for heart transplantation; the grafts in this group did not survive. A third group received a heavier immunosuppression regimen comprised of tacrolimus, prednisolone, and mycophenolate mofetil. The survival of grafts two months post-transplant for this group was 100 percent. These findings are a clear indication that HLA banking does not avoid the risk of rejection and antigen recognition, which subsequently leads to rejection and loss of the grafts, Schrepfer stated.

## Hypoimmune Cell Products: Protecting Allogenic Cells from Immune Destruction

The beauty of stem cell–based therapy is the accessibility of cells and the longer time frame during which they can be modified, Schrepfer remarked. Whereas solid organs have a short window of approximately six hours in which to be transplanted, researchers have time to modify stem cells and iPSCs. If researchers can utilize gene editing tools on iPSCs from healthy donors to create hypoimmune cell products, these could be available off the shelf for any patient. Advantages of such technology over other approaches are considerable, she said (see Box 4-1). Cells that are truly hypoimmune eliminate the need for immunosuppression treatment to avoid immune rejection. A well-characterized master cell line could be developed from one healthy donor, avoiding the need for cumbersome banking of huge numbers of cell lines and enabling easier manufacturing and quality control, Schrepfer explained.

### Adaptive and Innate Immune Responses to Human Leukocyte Antigen in Allogeneic Cells

The field of hypoimmunity started years ago when researchers began studying a naturally occurring allogeneic graft—the fetus in a pregnant

---

**BOX 4-1**
**Advantages of Hypoimmune Cell Products**

- No immune rejection
  - Evades allogeneic immune rejection
  - Does not activate the "missing self" response from natural killer cells and macrophages
- No need to generate individualized cell products
- No cumbersome banking of huge amounts of cell lines
- One well-characterized master cell line
- Easier manufacturing and quality control
- Ample availability of cell products
- Can be transplanted into sensitized recipients
- Do not alter the recipient's immune system

SOURCE: Schrepfer presentation, November 2, 2021.

mother, said Schrepfer. Half of fetal proteins are from the father, and the mother's immune system recognizes the proteins as allogeneic (i.e., foreign) yet does not reject the fetus. Schrepfer and colleagues in the field studied feto–maternal immune tolerance, including molecules that are upregulated and downregulated, in an effort to understand the combination of molecules that could create a hypoimmune cell product. This concept of hypoimmune is an alternative approach to overcoming the immune barrier; hypoimmunity differs from tolerance induction in that it is based on the idea of immune evasion, whereby the immune system does not recognize the cell product after transplantation, Schrepfer noted. Adaptive immunity presents a major challenge in cellular transplantation (see Figure 4-2). When T cells recognize the HLA molecules of allogeneic cells, they kill and reject those cells. Researchers have come to understand that HLA removal overcomes the T-cell response. However, HLAs also inhibit other cell types, such as natural killer (NK) cells, that are part of the innate immune system. Thus, removing the HLAs introduces a new issue to allogeneic transplantation—that is, killing by innate immune cells.

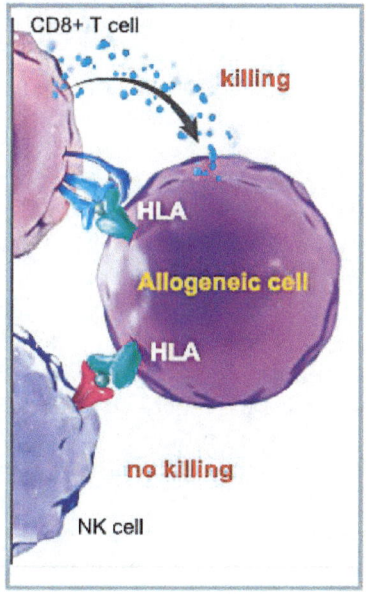 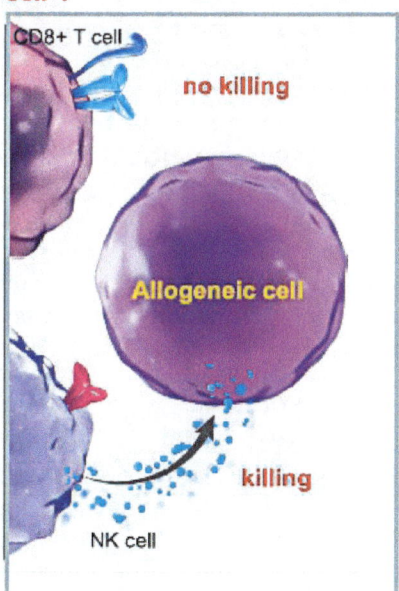

**FIGURE 4-2** Adaptive and innate immune responses to allogeneic cells.
NOTE: HLA = human leukocyte antigen; NK = natural killer.
SOURCE: Schrepfer presentation, November 2, 2021.

*Molecules to Prevent Killing of HLA-knockout Target Cells by Innate Immune Response*

Researchers are investigating potential molecules that, when overexpressed, are hypothesized to inhibit innate immune cell killing. Schrepfer and colleagues tested the separate effects of overexpression of four molecules—HLA-E, HLA-G, programmed death-ligand 1, and CD47—using a cell line that does not express HLAs and was cultured with NK cells. When the assay was conducted with primary NK cells, such as those found in the human body, most of the molecules were not able to prevent the NK cell population from activating and killing the allogeneic cells. The CD47 molecule, however, can inhibit both subpopulations of NK cells and the entire NK cell population in a human body. With the creation of hypoimmune cells as a genetic endpoint, the engineering approach to off-the-shelf cell therapies involves taking iPSCs from healthy donors, removing HLA class I and II molecules, and then overexpressing CD47 (Deuse et al., 2021a; Deuse et al., 2019; Deuse et al., 2021b; Hu et al., 2021). The goal of creating off-the-shelf therapies is to eliminate the need for immunosuppression and to have these therapies available for anyone, at anytime, anywhere, Schrepfer highlighted.

Recent research has demonstrated that this method not only overcomes the allogeneic barrier but also enables the transplantation of fully functional cells. Researchers differentiated iPSCs from mice into endothelial cells and found that in T-cell activation assays of unmodified endothelial cells, allogeneic activation of T cells was much higher than in syngeneic transplantation, a process in which immune rejection is not expected (Deuse et al., 2019). Similarly, in subsequent antibody binding, immunoglobulin M (IgM) antibodies were higher in allogeneic activated samples than in syngeneic transplants. However, for hypoimmune endothelial cells, T-cell activation and IgM antibodies were similar for allogeneic activation and syngeneic transplantation (Deuse et al., 2019). Furthermore, studies in a disease model for hind-limb ischemia in mice showed that the unmodified, wild-type endothelial cells died and the hypoimmune cells survived (Deuse et al., 2021b). The animals injected with wild-type iPSC-derived endothelial cells experienced limb loss. In contrast, the hypoimmune iPSC-derived endothelial cells not only survived but also restored vascularization in mice that received them without immunosuppression (Deuse et al., 2021b). The goal of regenerative therapy extends beyond overcoming the immune barrier to enable cells to function as intended in vivo, Schrepfer emphasized.

### Immunosuppression-Free Future of Regenerative Therapies

Nonhuman-primate (NHP) studies set a high bar for immune studies, because the NHP immune system is so active, Schrepfer noted. Researchers found that when unmodified iPSCs were injected into monkeys, T-cell activation was high. However, transplanted hypoimmune iPSCs avoided immune system detection and antibody production in allogeneic NHP recipients. She noted that immune evasion was achieved even after prior sensitization in monkeys, an important finding given that regenerative medicine should consider the needs of sensitized patients who may require redosing, or repetitive treatment. Researchers also found in NHPs that the CD47 molecule prevents the killing of hypoimmune iPSCs; the cells will survive when CD47 is present but are killed when CD47 is blocked. Finally, the unmodified iPSCs were rejected in rhesus monkeys after three weeks, whereas the hypoimmune iPSCs survived. When all immune system components are considered—NK cells as well as T cells—immune evasion with hypoimmune cells appears to be an achievable goal, Schrepfer said.

Schrepfer was optimistic that the future of regenerative therapies could be immunosuppression free, given that cellular transplantation without immunosuppression appears to be achievable using hypoimmune cells. Together, the findings she presented show that hypoimmune cells (1) evade allogeneic immune rejection; (2) do not activate the "missing self" response from NK cells and macrophages; (3) can be transplanted into sensitized recipients, offering the possibility of redosing; and (4) do not alter the recipient's immune system (Box 4-1).

## OFF-THE-SHELF ENGINEERED IPSC-DERIVED NATURAL KILLER AND T CELLS FOR THE TREATMENT OF CANCER

Bob Valamehr, chief research and development officer at Fate Therapeutics, provided an overview of his company's cell therapy platform. Although the iPSC-derived off-the-shelf platform is novel, the Fate Therapeutics approach provides similar benefits to more conventional strategies and drug development. The process begins with a starting material that is uniform and consistent for manufacture; in this case, the starting material is a master cell bank. The key reagent is a stem cell that has been highly engineered, banked, and fully characterized, he explained. Consistent starting material enables mass production of the cell type of choice. Multiple cell types can be made from stem cells, including NK and T cells. Mass production now allows the creation of a uniform product that is frozen in bags and ready to be shipped to hospitals. The frozen material can be thawed and directly infused, representing a new treatment paradigm in cell therapy, in which treatment is available on demand and provided in outpatient settings, he explained.

### Off-the-Shelf Cell Therapy Platform

At the heart of the master cell bank are iPSCs, which can be made into any of the 200 cell types found in the body, said Valamehr. When these cells are properly maintained, they have unlimited self-renewal capacity. Changing the culture conditions enables the cells to differentiate. For instance, Fate Therapeutics has been working on hematopoietic cell lineage differentiation, and they have established control over the cells to the extent that they are now able to dissociate iPSCs into single cells. Those individual cells are engineered to expand a uniform population of multi-edited engineered products (see Figure 4-3). The uniform composition and fully characterized master cell bank enable a renewable clonal cell line that can be used to create homogenous cell products. Valamehr explained that iPSCs are first edited, individual cells are allowed to expand into clonal populations, and then researchers compare individual clones for desired attributes. Screening occurs at both the molecular and functional level to select for desired attributes and avoid undesired traits, such as off-target editing or genomic instability. Thousands of clones are screened to select an individual clone that is then used to create a master cell bank. This renewable starting material can be used to make high-quality NK and T cells that are frozen in bags, delivered, thawed, and directly infused in outpatient settings. This off-the-shelf platform allows for multiplex engineering of a homogenous product, mass production, and off-the-shelf cell therapy application, he said.

*Developing Novel Multiplexed Engineered Cells with*
*Multi-Antigen Specificity*

Ongoing work at Fate Therapeutics aims to develop novel multiplexed engineered iNK and iT cells with multi-antigen specificity to combat tumor heterogeneity and treatment resistance. Multiple components can be edited into a cell to create highly effective effector cells, Valamehr explained, and Fate Therapeutics focuses on multiple attributes in producing high-quality NK and T cells. He remarked that cancer is smart, and therefore it must be attacked in a multipronged manner. This involves putting multiple targeting entities onto the cell that enable the cell to attack the target through chimeric antigen receptor (CAR) T-cell receptor, CD16 receptor, and other novel strategies. For instance, cells are targeted to attack antigens specific to cancer. Once targeting entities are added to the cell, the cell product is combined with other effective therapeutic agents, such as monoclonal antibodies, checkpoint blockade therapy, T and NK cell engagers, and radiation

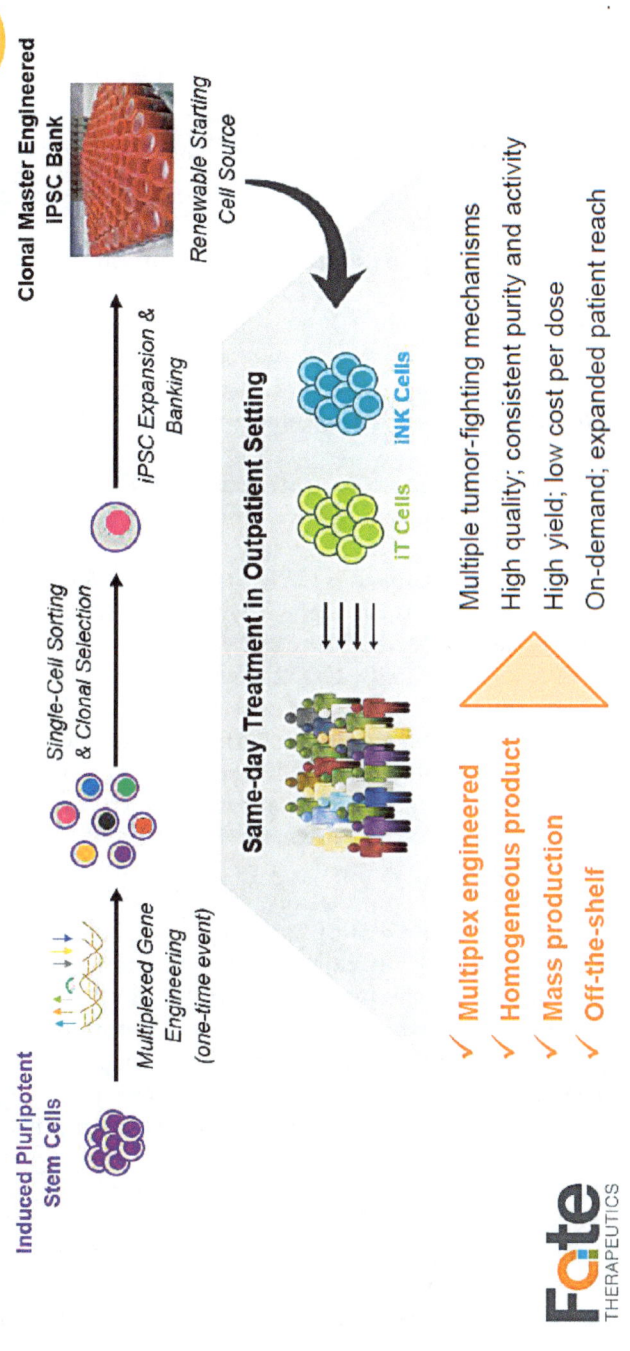

**FIGURE 4-3** Platform for mass production of induced pluripotent stem cell products.
NOTE: iPSC = induced pluripotent stem cell; NK = natural killer.
SOURCE: Valamehr presentation, November 2, 2021.

therapy (Saetersmoen et al., 2019). The manufacturing of NK and T cells allows different effector cells to be combined to introduce both innate and adaptive immunity into a patient, Valamehr explained.

## Chimeric Antigen Receptor T-Cell Therapy

Fate Therapeutics is focusing their pipeline on CAR-targeting strategies, Valamehr said. The pipeline consists of multifaceted, multi-targeted CAR T and NK cells that can be synergized with current therapeutic agents. A CAR-19 NK therapy—dubbed FT596—that targets CD19 for B-cell malignancies is currently in clinical trials. This novel dual-antigen targeting strategy of FT596 is designed to overcome tumor heterogeneity and antigen escape for a durable response in B-cell malignancies. FT596 is an NK cell containing three specific antitumor modalities (Woan et al., 2021); the first is a high-affinity noncleavable CD16 (hnCD16) that maximizes antibody-dependent cell-mediated cytotoxicity (ADCC) (Jing et al., 2015). The modality hnCD16 enables effective elimination by engaging with the antibody, which in turn engages with the cancer cell (Zhu et al., 2020). The second antitumor modality is a CAR that targets CD19 and facilitates targeting of multiple antigens on a given lymphoma (Li et al., 2018). For instance, the CAR that targets CD19 can be combined with a monoclonal antibody (mAb) targeting CD20, CD22, or CD123. Third, FT596 has an interleukin (IL)-15 receptor fusion that causes NK cells to be more resilient and persistent, enabling them to survive without endogenous cytokine support (Woan et al., 2021). Typically, NK cells are challenging to engineer because they respond to the input of a transgene by expelling it, said Valamehr. However, since it starts from a clonal population of engineered iPSCs, the Fate Therapeutics final product is a pure population of NK cells—as defined by the CD45/CD56 population—that carries uniform expression of CARs and CD16. A single vial of banked starting material can produce over 1 trillion iPSC-derived NK cells, and by expanding the volume from 100 liters to 10,000 liters, the number of produced NK cells can increase to 100 trillion. Preclinical studies indicate that a multidose application of FT596 controls the NALM6 cell line in mice, Valamehr said.

The clinical protocol for FT596 tested the treatment on B-cell lymphoma as a monotherapy and in combination with rituximab. The chemotherapy cyclophosphamide was used to make space for the FT596 by eliminating immune cells through lympho-conditioning and lympho-depletion. Cyclophosphamide also increases homeostatic cytokines in the body. Furthermore, this drug rids the environment of CD8, CD4 cells, or NK cells that could potentially eliminate FT596 in the allogeneic setting. After cyclophosphamide treatment, one dose of FT596 was given either as a monotherapy or in combination with rituximab. The treatment was assessed 29 days later, and the study found that FT596 demonstrated dose-dependent efficacy. A dose of 30 million cells did not indicate clinical response. However, patients responded to single doses of 90 million and 300 million cells administered as fourth or fifth lines of therapy. FT596 is one of the first off-the-shelf iPSC-derived products in an allogeneic setting that shows antitumor activity and contribution to disease control, Valamehr remarked. Of the 14 patients tested, 10 achieved overall response and 7 achieved complete response.

### Strategies for Evading the Immune System

The three approaches Fate Therapeutics uses to evade the host immune system include cloak, eliminate, and attack and proliferate, Valamehr outlined. The cloaking strategy involves knocking out genes associated with CD8, CD4, and NK cell engagement. This process cloaks the product from detection by dismissing engagement of T and NK cells with the cell product. The elimination strategy utilizes mAb CD38 to eliminate activated effector cells found in the body. When T and NK cells are activated, they express CD38; therefore, daratumumab, an anti-CD38 mAb, is administered to a patient with hnCD16 to eliminate any activated NK or T cells in the vicinity, Valamehr explained. The product avoids self-destruction because it is a CD38 knockout, while still supporting the killing of other activated cells that come near it. The final strategy of attack and proliferation utilizes an alloimmune defense strategy designed for patients with treatment regimens that do not include cyclophosphamide (Mo et al., 2021). A novel synthetic receptor eliminates nearby alloreactive immune cells and simultaneously provides a biological signal to promote positive cellular proliferation. This product not only survives in the host immune system, but it also becomes activated through engagement with the host immune system, Valamehr remarked. Fate Therapeutics is advancing both these novel immune evasion strategies and off-the-shelf T and NK cell products, which may be combined to combat cancer and its process of evolution, he said.

## DISCUSSION

### Cell Therapy Risk Mitigation

A member of the community asked Schrepfer and Valamehr how to mitigate the risk of engineered cells becoming malignant or out of control. The safety aspects of cellular transplants that evade immune recognition must be considered, Schrepfer replied. One concern is the possibility that viral load could lead to HLA-negative cells becoming infected. The risk of that occurring is yet to be determined, and it merits further research, especially when considering that knockout mice have been able to clear viruses, she stated. Another concern is that, theoretically, iPSCs carry the risk of teratoma formation. Furthermore, the cells may not function as they are designed to function, and mitigating risk involves controlling for that. Control is not only needed for immune evasion strategies but also for tolerance induction approaches, she added. Should something go awry in a setting of tolerance induction, such as an insulin-producing beta cell not functioning as it should, a safety backup may be required. Beyond overcoming immune barriers and avoiding cell rejection, strategies to control the cells are needed as well as research on the benefits and risks for specific patient populations, said Schrepfer.

The beauty of off-the-shelf products is that they can be highly characterized, Valamehr remarked. Before a developed product is administered to a patient, it is studied for months to determine standard dosage, the maximal dosage that would ever be reached, and tumor toxicity. The product is fully characterized for genomic stability, in vitro oncogenicity, and safety perspectives in the tumor toxicity study. Whereas the critical mission of an autologous treatment is administration to the patient, the off-the-shelf setting allows for thorough testing to enable confidence that the product will not revert, has no residuals, and is effective, said Valamehr.

Salzman asked the speakers whether generation methods for making iPSCs can cause mutations in mitochondria and, if so, whether that potential problem can be mitigated. Mutations are dependent on how cells are handled; for instance, freezing and thawing increases the risk of mutation, Schrepfer responded. Processes can be optimized to build quality control by analyzing mutations and methods that increase risk, she added. At the center of Fate Therapeutics' strategy is screening clones, Valamehr noted. By screening 1,000 clones, researchers can detect undesired effects and changes in the host mitochondrial genome. Over the course of multiple years, they follow the entire development of the clone and establish deep familiarity with it. Clone selection provides options of different attributes that can be selected or deselected to avoid undesirable mutations, he said. It is different with MSCs since they are natural cells and are limited by nature, Le Blanc added.

## Mesenchymal Stromal Cell Therapy

Given that most MSC products are approved for local injection rather than infusion, Salzman asked Le Blanc about the risk–benefit profile of MSCs and how this applies on a translational level. There may be more safety data on infusion delivery than on local delivery, and these safety data are extraordinary, Le Blanc responded. It is rare for a treatment to have as few side effects as does intravenous injection of MSCs; however, efficacy has not been achieved thus far, she added. Furthermore, greater understanding is needed regarding who should be targeted with MSCs. Drawing a parallel to a scenario in which all fever patients are treated with penicillin despite the fact that not all fevers are caused by penicillin-sensitive bacteria, she stated that the biology of disease should be better understood in order to target treatment appropriately. Salzman added that the opportunity for a perfect solution seems to lie in finding a treatment that provides the right amount of benefit—neither too little nor too much—while avoiding high risk.

Since MHC concerns do not apply to MSCs, Salzman asked Le Blanc whether MSCs are created alike or if variability is found across a population in terms of external profiling. Salzman asked how wide the spectrum of variability among donor MSCs is in contrast to hematopoietic stem cells or other cell sources. MSCs do not engraft and instead disappear in the blood stream within minutes, Le Blanc replied. She posited that rapid destruction is more likely at play than pure rejection or lack of engraftment. This is seen in local injection in the vocal fold system. The vocal fold is a fairly immune privileged site, yet MSCs are not found a day or two after injection. Immune responses have been detected, but these are minor, and true rejection is therefore unlikely to be the cause of the rapid disappearance of cells, she said.

## Specifics of Hypoimmunity

Salzman asked Schrepfer about the stage of cell development at which the effects of engineered hypoimmunity become apparent in stem cells such as iPSCs, embryonic stem cells (ESCs), mesoderm, and hematopoietic stem cells. Schrepfer replied that when she entered the field in 2005, many researchers hoped that ESCs—and later iPSCs—held the potential to evade detection by the immune system due to their early stage of development, therefore these cells or their derivatives could be transplanted into anyone without immune recognition. The current understanding is that regardless of the state, the HLAs and the alloantigens they present will eventually be recognized by the immune system. Thus, no cell state protects against immune recognition and subsequent rejection, she said. Another concept focuses on the transplant site rather than on the cell. Some researchers believe that certain sites, such as the brain and eye, may be immunoprivileged. Cell transplantation typically breaks the blood–brain barrier, resulting in the immunoprivileged organ losing its immune privilege, she explained. Clinical practices must therefore consider the handling of tissue and the environment. Schrepfer stated that she does not think tissues, organs, or allogenic cells are immune privileged, although some cell types such as MSCs have immune-privileged capabilities. Despite this, the risk of MSCs being recognized and rejected in an allogenic setting persists.

Given that CD47 is known to emit a signal directing macrophages not to eat the cells, Schrepfer was asked whether overexpression of CD47 inhibits phagocytosis-mediated clearance of apoptotic donor cells by tissue-resident macrophages. While CD47 is known as the "don't eat me" protein, Schrepfer calls it the "don't kill me" protein because it also works on NK cells with a different mechanism than the one it utilizes on macrophages. Necrotic and apoptotic cells will still be cleared when CD47 is overexpressed because the molecules are no longer functional and are therefore unable to prevent cell clearance. Some cell death will occur during cell transplantation due to the stress of the process and the lack of oxygen, and dead cells need to be cleared. Apoptosis and necrosis render the molecules unable to inhibit clearance by macrophages, she explained.

Salzman also asked Schrepfer about the barriers involved in the placenta during pregnancy and how barriers may be used to generate hypoimmunity. Pregnancy is unique and fetal–maternal tolerance does not translate directly to hypoimmunity, Schrepfer replied. Pregnancy involves the inhibition of various immune populations at different times. For instance, high numbers of Tregs are needed during implantation of the fetus, but not later in pregnancy. Schrepfer and her colleagues have used the concept of pregnancy in studying the effects of molecules on immune populations. The barrier from fetus to mother is open, allowing for the trafficking of immune cells. Unfortunately, this process cannot be translated to cell transplantation, but the concept is used to start understanding the molecules involved, she said.

### Strategies for Evading the Immune System

Valamehr was asked by a community member to speculate about which of the Fate Therapeutics' strategies is best suited for transplants versus short-term use of iPSCs, such as immune cell therapy. The strategies of elimination and of attack and proliferation are only for cells that have the ability to kill, Valamehr replied. Eliciting an ADCC or CAR response is reserved for transient effector cells. The first strategy of cloaking breaks engagement and is used for regenerative medicine. He noted that other approaches exist beyond those that utilize T and NK cells, and he and his colleagues are working on a strategy that will disengage all interactions.

### Expansion of Cellular Therapy Distribution

Salzman asked Valamehr about processes for dosing and repeat dosing off-the-shelf products and about the next frontier in off-the-shelf cell therapy. Distributing cell products into community hospitals is the next goal, he replied. Few people live near a cellular therapy research facility, and therefore distributing products into as many locations as possible will increase the reach of therapeutic benefit to more people. Fate Therapeutics currently has two manufacturing sites and is planning to grow their manufacturing capacity. Ideally, patients will eventually be able to go to a pharmacy or local hospital and have the prescribed product thawed and administered on an outpatient basis in the community setting. He added that an overall goal is to enable multidosing. Just as aspirin can be taken every four hours until a headache goes away, cellular therapy could be administered until desired results are achieved. Currently, at low-scale production, each dose costs less than $5,000. Valamehr described a vision in which everyone has access to cellular therapy administered in a multidose manner until the cancer is gone.

## Patient Profiling and Conditioning

Salzman asked Valemehr to elaborate on the benefits of conditioning patients before cell therapy and whether pathways in the future may eliminate the burden of conditioning on the patient. Conditioning in a cancer setting serves multiple purposes, Valamehr replied. Conditioning acts as an antitumor agent and creates space for the cell therapy. Competition within the body for cytokines limits available space in bone marrow. Conditioning allows for reducing endogenous immune cells, CD8s, CD4s, and NK cells that may reject the product while increasing homeostatic cytokines such as IL15. These effects hold value while simultaneously depleting the host immune system. FT596 has been administered in doses containing up to 900 million cells without being rejected, albeit in a population of cancer patients with exhausted immune systems, Valamehr noted. In a situation involving a solid tumor where the product is being used as frontline treatment, light conditioning is preferred to traditional conditioning. This involves creating a setting in which the product can work in concert with and take advantage of the endogenous immune system and induce a second wave of immunity. CAR therapy relies heavily on cyclophosphamide, but strategies involving allodefense receptors may overcome the need for conditioning in the future, said Valamehr.

Given that various patient profiles respond differently to treatment, Salzman asked the speakers what aspects of the target product profile should be considered and how the cell product could best match the profile of a patient experiencing an unmet health need. Schrepfer responded that researchers must consider that each disease is different, each patient has different viral infections, and that the immune system needs to be in a certain state in order to establish tolerance. In contrast, immune evasion does not require a specific immune system status because the goal of this concept is to completely avoid cell recognition. Because evasion overcomes the need for the patient to have a certain immune state, evasion complements tolerance therapies, she added. Many clinical diagnoses of inflammatory disorders are made based on symptoms rather than on biology, Le Blanc remarked. Including biology in both staging and diagnosing disease will shed light on treatment requirements, she reiterated. Valamehr commented on the importance of universality and multi-antigen targeting. Targeting a cancer in multiple ways and targeting the immune system will enable cancer patients to be treated and to persist long enough to receive benefit from the treatments.

# 5

# Endogenous Regeneration and the Role of the Local Environment in Repair

> **Key Points Highlighted by Individual Speakers**
>
> - Aging involves loss of muscle mass and strength, regulated by an essential "pro-inflammatory" metabolite called prostaglandin E2 (PGE2) and its degrading enzyme 15-hydroxyprostaglandin dehydrogenase (15-PGDH). (Blau)
> - PGE2 is associated with greater muscle mass, strength, and endurance. 15-PGDH is an enzyme that degrades PGE2 and is a hallmark of aged tissues. Decreases in 15-PGDH increase PGE2. (Blau)
> - B cells can have two different roles in the wound environment depending on their maturity and the timing of their recruitment. Immature B cells promote healing; mature B cells are associated with fibrosis. (Moore)
> - Developmental endothelial locus-1 (DEL-1) is a secreted protein with many functions and potential therapeutic implications. Depending on its location, DEL-1 can regulate neutrophil recruitment, promote inflammation resolution, or induce bone regeneration. (Hajishengallis)
> - Endogenous opportunities for healing might be leveraged to enhance effectiveness of other therapies or overcome negative effects of aging. (Blau, Hajishengallis, Moore)
> - Timing of intervention is a significant factor in the strategic modulation of wound healing and regenerative responses. (Moore)

The objectives of the third session of the workshop were to (1) examine what "proper healing" looks like at the level of the local environment and discuss relevant research gaps and (2) consider the effects of aging, gender, and other variables and pathological changes on the local environment, endogenous repair, and wound healing. Steven Becker, program director of the Structural Biology and Molecular Applications Branch at the National Cancer Institute at the time of the workshop, moderated the session.

## REVERSING AGING: PRO-INFLAMMATORY METABOLITE PROSTAGLANDIN E2 AUGMENTS MUSCLE REGENERATION

Helen Blau, Donald E. and Delia B. Baxter Foundation Professor and director of the Baxter Laboratory for Stem Cell Biology at Stanford University, discussed the discovery that prostaglandin E2 (PGE2), an inflammatory metabolite, is crucial to muscle regeneration. PGE2 also plays a major role in aging, and targeting its degradation can both ameliorate aging and promote regeneration, effectively reversing the aging process in muscle, she said. Regenerative medicine questions whether aging must entail debility that hampers quality of life in old age, Blau observed. Life expectancy has increased over the past 15 years for both men and women (Bellantuono, 2018). However, it is life span—rather than healthspan—that is increasing, so people spend more years living with chronic disease. Men born in 2014 are expected to experience three more years with chronic disease than are those born in 2006. Blau highlighted the goal of improving quality of life and healthspan through regenerative medicine.

### Combating Muscle Wasting

Muscle supports a high quality of life because it is central to all life activities, from dancing in a ballet to using diaphragm muscles while sitting, said Blau. Aging can involve a devastating loss of muscle mass and strength, where the average human loses 10 percent of their muscle mass per decade after the age of 50 (Hunt et al., 2015). One third of the population aged 80 years or older is affected by the debilitating loss of muscle mass and strength known as sarcopenia (Looker and Wang, 2015). Loss of muscle mass has severe consequences (Burns et al., 2016). As people become frail, they are less able to perform everyday tasks, including walking and rising from a chair. Falls become more common, resulting in $31 billion in annual injury treatment costs for nonfatal falls (Burns et al., 2016). As tasks of daily living become more difficult, people become more dependent and may require institutionalization, which carries further high health care costs. Sarcopenia is also associated with increased mortality, Blau noted.

Muscle stem cells (MuSCs) are essential to muscle regeneration, and they give rise to two key methods to combat muscle wasting, including (1) MuSC stimulation to enhance regeneration and (2) muscle myofiber rejuvenation, Blau explained. Both approaches are mediated by the metabolite PGE2. MuSCs are resident in muscle tissue and are dedicated to the repair of muscle throughout life. Located in niches along the basal lamina of the myofiber, MuSCs are in a quiescent state until injury occurs. When the muscle is injured, the stem cells are activated and express myoblast determination protein 1, also known as MyoD. The MuSCs then become committed progenitors that express fusion proteins that mediate fusion with the damaged myofibers, replenishing them with new nuclei and, consequently, new DNA. Interestingly, this is the same population of stem cells which Alexander Mauro correctly postulated that he saw on electron micrographs and which he referred to as satellite cells in 1961, Blau noted (Mauro, 1961).

## Effect of Prostaglandin E2 on Muscle Repair

A natural inflammatory regulator, PGE2 is one of the body's first responses to injury. Injury triggers waves of sequential cellular activity, beginning with inflammation, followed by fibroadipocytes and fibroblasts and then by activation of MuSCs. Blau and her team reasoned that a regulator in this cascade must strongly influence the function of MuSCs and that aging alters this effect (Blau et al., 2015). Andrew Ho and Adelaida Palla, scientists from the Baxter Laboratory for Stem Cell Biology at Stanford University, conducted a bioinformatic analysis of the transcriptome of activated stem cells acutely post-injury (Ho et al., 2017). They culled a common gene list of activated MuSC transcripts and used Ingenuity Pathway Analysis to focus on transmembrane and receptor genes (Ho et al., 2017). Ho and Palla identified EP4, an E-type prostanoid receptor for PGE2, as one of the most common receptors in the category of inflammation, suggesting an important role for PGE2 in stimulating MuSC function and repair. Despite its important role, PGE2 may be understudied because it is a metabolite and would, therefore, not appear on a transcriptome, Blau explained. PGE2 is derived from arachidonic acid via several enzymatic steps. Although PGE2 can work on any one of four EP receptors, EP4 is by far the most prevalent in MuSCs and muscle fibers, and EP4 signals through cyclic adenosine monophosphate (cAMP) (Ho et al., 2017). In addition, nonsteroidal anti-inflammatory drugs (NSAIDs) such as indomethacin and ibuprofen block cyclooxygenase enzymes (COX-1 and -2), which in turn block the endogenous synthesis of PGE2 after injury, Blau noted (Ho et al., 2017).

*Loss of Prostaglandin E2 Signaling in Muscle Stem Cells
Impairs Muscle Regeneration*

To determine whether this pathway is crucial to the function of MuSCs, Blau and her colleagues conducted a conditional genetic ablation of the receptor EP4 on MuSCs in a mouse model using the promoter of paired box 7 (PAX7), a transcription factor that is a hallmark of the stem cell and drives floxing of EP4 in the knockout model. The researchers performed an injury by injecting notexin, a snake venom toxin commonly used in the field to cause muscle injury. Several weeks later, strength was measured using a foot pedal measurement of displacement. They found that when the stem cells could not sense PGE2 due to a lack of EP4 receptors, the mice experienced a 50 percent decrease in strength, both in twitch force and tetanic force (Ho et al., 2017). Therefore, this pathway is extremely important for enabling stem cells to proliferate, expand, and repair the damage, and young mice became weaker after injury due to their inability to repair muscle damage, Blau explained.

*NSAID Treatment Decreases Endogenous Prostaglandin E2
Signaling after Injury and Impairs Muscle Strength*

Blau and her team further examined the role of PGE2 signaling through loss-of-function experiments. For instance, using another mouse model with PAX7-driven luciferase expression, they performed a muscle injury and administered an NSAID, the equivalent of an ibuprofen injection (Ho et al., 2017). Reduced bioluminescence, a readout of luciferase, correlates with fewer stem cells due to decreased proliferation and expansion in comparison to mice that did not receive the NSAID, Blau described. Twitch force also saw a remarkable decline, she noted. *The New York Times* highlighted this study in an article entitled "Bring on the Exercise, Hold the Painkillers" (Reynolds, 2017). Although many people take ibuprofen after working out to decrease achiness, taking an NSAID negates the benefit of exercise, and the injury associated with exercise is part of building muscle and muscle strength, Blau remarked. The pathway is essential to proper stem cell function, and if PGE2 signaling is blocked, the cells lose much of their ability to divide, repair injury, and build strength, she said.

### Globally Increasing Muscle Function with Prostaglandin E2

Their findings about the local effects of PGE2 led Blau and her colleagues to wonder whether global PGE2 levels could be increased and what effect that would have on muscle function. While working at the Baxter Laboratory for Stem Cell Biology at Stanford University,

Adelaida Palla, Meenakshi Ravichandran, and Yu Xin Wang discovered that 15-hydroxyprostaglandin dehydrogenase (15-PGDH), the degrading enzyme of PGE2, is a novel molecular determinant of muscle aging and a regulator of prostaglandins that is crucial to muscle function (Palla et al., 2021). Furthermore, they found that 15-PGDH is a hallmark of aging and can be targeted for rejuvenation. Given the muscle weakness associated with aging, Blau and her team reasoned that PGE2 might decline with age. By measuring levels of PGE2 and prostaglandin D2 (PGD2) by mass spectrometry, they found that these metabolites decreased by approximately 30 percent with aging (Palla et al., 2021). They hypothesized that this decline might result from an elevation in the enzyme that degrades these prostaglandins. Indeed, a comparison of 15-PGDH levels in young and aged mouse tissues revealed that the enzyme not only increased in aged muscle, but also in the colon, spleen, skin, and heart (Palla et al., 2021). Thus, 15-PGDH appears to be a hallmark of aging in multiple tissues. The researchers also mined a publicly available microarray database for 15-PGDH expression to determine whether their finding held for human tissue, and they discovered higher levels of the enzyme in aged humans as well (Palla et al., 2021). Blau noted that 15-PGDH expression—like all hallmarks of aging—is on a spectrum, with some people being biologically younger than their peers.

To test whether targeting the degradation enzyme, 15-PGDH, would increase PGE2 levels, researchers used a small molecule inhibitor, SW033291, and administered daily intraperitoneal injections of the inhibitor to aged mice for one month, Blau explained. This resulted in the degrading enzyme, 15-PGDH, decreasing by approximately 30 percent and a consequent two-fold increase in PGE2 and PGD2, constituting a return to youthful levels (Palla et al., 2021). The inhibition of 15-PGDH and the resulting increase of PGE2 were associated with a significant increase in muscle mass in the gastrocnemius, tibialis anterior, and soleus muscles, and therefore had an effect on both fast- and slow-contracting muscle types (Palla et al., 2021). Furthermore, muscle strength and force relative to baseline also increased in both young and aged mice. Moreover, endurance, measured by time to exhaustion on a treadmill, also significantly increased, which presumably involves more than simply skeletal muscle, remarked Blau. In order to ensure that these results were specific to 15-PGDH, the experiment was replicated using a genetic knockdown of 15-PGDH with a short hairpin RNA, and the same results were found with increases in muscle mass, muscle strength, and force relative to baseline (Palla et al., 2021). Utilizing CO-Detection by indEXing (CODEX) imaging, Blau's team found that myofibers and macrophages were the source of 15-PGDH in aging. Accordingly, the researchers overexpressed this enzyme in young mouse models, and muscle mass, strength, and force declined within a month. Remarkably, muscles shrank and weakened in response to overexpression of a single enzyme, Blau emphasized. When

15-PGDH increased, PGE2 and PGD2 decreased, further validating earlier findings. These experiments demonstrate that 15-PGDH is a pivotal regulator of aging and rejuvenation, she said.

### 15-PGDH Inhibition Mechanism of Action

To determine the mechanism responsible for 15-PGDH inhibition, Blau and colleagues compared heatmaps of gene expression for three vehicle-treated mice and three mice treated with a small molecule inhibitor (SW033291) for one month (Palla et al., 2021). The mice injected with SW033291 showed a marked down-regulation of ubiquitin ligases, which are enzymes responsible for protein degradation in aging muscle. Researchers also found a decline in transforming growth factor beta (TGF-beta) signaling, including myostatin, which is a common target of therapeutics pursued in biotechnology and pharmaceutical companies for attempting to increase muscle mass (Palla et al., 2021). The results suggest that PGE2 is upstream of myostatin and that inhibition of the enzyme 15-PGDH inhibits deleterious pathways responsible for muscle degradation, Blau explained. These findings were also validated by polymerase chain reaction (PCR) testing, she noted. In addition, researchers found that inhibiting 15-PGDH spurred an increase in mitochondrial function. Heatmaps of gene expression indicated dramatic upregulation of mitochondria-related gene expression, the effects of which can be observed on an electron micrograph. Aged mouse muscle tissue featured distended, vacuous, dysfunctional mitochondria. After aged mice received one month of treatment, muscle tissue was remodeled to a youthful structure with intact myofibrils and condensed mitochondria in orderly pairs, described Blau. Quantitative analysis revealed that the autophagy protein p62 increased with treatment and is likely largely responsible for promoting mitochondrial biogenesis and restoring mitochondrial function. Additionally, an examination of Krebs cycle components indicated that citrate synthase, succinate dehydrogenase, and membrane potential all decline with aging and are restored with 15-PGDH inhibition treatment. Therefore, inhibiting the degrading enzyme restored mitochondrial function, increased mitochondrial numbers, and improved function in electron transfer and energy production, she added.

Blau concluded by emphasizing that (1) prostaglandin signaling is critical for muscle maintenance, regeneration, and rejuvenation and (2) a small molecule inhibitor of 15-PGDH has pleiotropic beneficial effects through enhancing PGE2. She provided an overview of key findings on the role of PGE2 on muscle fiber and MuSC function (see Box 5-1). PGE2 is an essential inflammatory metabolite that is required for MuSC expansion and engraftment. Inhibiting 15-PGDH enhances PGE2, rejuvenating myofibers and stem cells. Elevated 15-PGDH, a key degrading enzyme, is a novel

> **BOX 5-1**
> **Key Research Findings on the Role of Prostaglandin Signaling in Muscle Function**
>
> Prostaglandin E2 (PGE2) augments muscle stem cell (MuSC) function:
> - PGE2 is an essential inflammatory metabolite for muscle regeneration via MuSCs—the body's natural healing mechanism.
> - PGE2 is required and sufficient for MuSC expansion and engraftment.
>
> PGE2 augments muscle fiber function:
> - 15-PGDH degrades PGE2 and is a novel hallmark of aged muscles and other aged tissues.
> - Benefit derives from physiologic modulation of inflammatory metabolite PGE2 to youthful levels.
> - Targeting 15-PGDH, a pivotal regulator of muscle aging, may be a therapeutic strategy to counter sarcopenia.
>
> SOURCE: Blau presentation, November 2, 2021.

hallmark of aging, and it can be targeted in a physiologic way. Modulating the levels of 15-PGDH twofold, to levels present in muscles of young mice, has a beneficial effect and holds therapeutic potential for countering sarcopenia and other conditions.

## BIOMATERIALS FOR MODELING IMMUNE MEDIATION IN WOUND HEALING

Erika Moore, Rhines Rising Star Larry Hench Assistant Professor at the University of Florida Department of Materials Science and Engineering, discussed the use of biomaterials for modeling immune cell mediation in wound healing. The inherent variability observed in wound healing creates an opportunity to use biomaterials to mimic differences in wound-healing environments. Minor injuries are typically met with pro-healing wound repair in which a small scar may be present but most tissue function is recovered, she explained. Conversely, dysregulated wound healing can result in keloid or hypertrophic scars. Pro-fibrotic wounds feature thick scar tissue and demonstrate the differentials that persist in wound healing. A patient-centered perspective would facilitate a better understanding of variability in wound healing because patients have different ancestral backgrounds, age contributors, experiences of trauma, and physical activity that can all contribute to the outcome in wound healing, Moore suggested.

## B-Cell Involvement in Wound Healing

To investigate variability in wound healing, Moore and her colleagues assessed immune cell coordination and contribution to the injury response. Multiple cell types orchestrate wound healing via cell-to-cell communications. B cells are known for their role in responding to vaccines and creating antibodies, enabling the immune system to recognize the antigen or stimulant in future exposures and develop an immune response against it; however, studying the role of B cells in wound healing is relatively controversial, Moore remarked. Yet, a previous study demonstrated that the presence or absence of B cells yielded differences in wound healing both early in the process and at subsequent points in the healing timeline (Iwata et al., 2009). In dermal skin wound injuries, B cells orchestrated healing in combination with other immune cells present at the site, resulting in more complete healing than in injuries in which B cells were absent (Iwata et al., 2009). These findings indicate that the role of B cells extends beyond antibody presentation and secretion to include critical involvement in wound healing, noted Moore. Furthermore, the dysregulation or dysfunction of B cells is associated with many diseases, including autoimmune disorders. She and her team sought to profile the connection between the immune response at the local tissue site and the systemic or whole-organism response and to learn how B cells operate during wound healing.

## Biomaterials to Manipulate Wound Healing

Moore and her team used biomaterials to create model systems of pro-healing and pro-fibrotic wounds to learn how B cells respond differently in these wound environments. In an effort to control the B-cell responses, the researchers leveraged biomaterial designs in mimicking wound-healing environments, utilizing pro-healing materials that promote wound healing or pro-fibrotic materials that encourage fibrosis or scar formation. Through these two types of biomaterials, the wound-healing process could be manipulated in order to assess the B-cell response in each of these environments, explained Moore. Researchers induced muscle injury in mice, implanted biomaterial directly into the wound, and interrogated the injury sites. In addition to interrogating the local response, they also examined both regional responses that included the lymph node and systemic responses that included the peritoneum and spleen. Moore emphasized that they sought to understand how the local environment and presence of specific biomaterials skew response toward healing or fibrosis and how that informs the entire systemic B-cell response.

The pro-healing materials promoted early recruitment of immature B cells to the wound sites, Moore said. In the control group, the average

B-cell count was below 5,000 on post-injury day 3 and slightly above 5,000 on day 5. In contrast, the average B-cell count in mice implanted with pro-healing material was above 10,000 on day 3 and increased to more than 15,000 on day 5 (a threefold increase over the injury control group) (Moore et al., 2021). Furthermore, the pro-healing materials promoted a regional response, with B cells generated at the local lymph nodes of the mice after injury. At one week post-injury, germinal centers had formed in the lymph nodes, indicating maturation of B cells in the mice implanted with pro-healing biomaterial. The generation of germinal centers did not appear in the control group or in the mice implanted with pro-fibrotic material, emphasized Moore. Therefore, the pro-healing material induced specific recognition and antigen response in B cells, beyond what occurs for injury alone.

Conversely, pro-fibrotic biomaterials were found to recruit mature B cells at later stages of wound healing, said Moore. Researchers studied the effects of mature B cells by conducting a B-cell knockout in mice and implanting pro-fibrotic biomaterial. Measurements of collagen and alpha-smooth muscle actin levels in mice with B cells indicated relatively high expression of these fibrosis-related markers. When scientists removed the mature B cells, the expression of both collagen and alpha-smooth muscle actin decreased (Moore et al., 2021). Thus, removing mature B cells reduced fibrosis and scar formation in the pro-fibrotic biomaterial environment, she stated.

## B Cells in Wound Healing

All people exist on a spectrum of healing, observed Moore. The ability to heal well is influenced by the tissue in which injury occurs, background, age, and other factors. This research is the first of its kind to test B-cell function in wound healing with the use of biomaterials, she remarked. Pro-healing materials were found to induce early recruitment of immature B cells, promoting healing. Pro-fibrotic materials recruited mature B cells, resulting in fibrosis. In turn, a reduction in fibrosis occurred with the removal of mature B cells from the injury site. Moore highlighted a dichotomy in the roles that B cells can play depending on their antigen-mature state, the maturity of the B cells, and on the timing of their recruitment to the injury site.

Moore and her colleagues investigate wound healing with the goal of achieving clinical relevance. One of those efforts is to study how B-cell response might alter or augment the body's acceptance of biomaterials implanted into breast tissue. Comparing human biopsies of patients implanted with naturally derived, pro-healing material with those of patients with silicone implants has revealed that the B-cell response differs in orientation and spread pattern between these two patient groups (see Figure 5-1). Understanding and classifying how biomaterials used in the clinic inform the immune response, and particularly the B-cell response, provides insight on the ability to regenerate, she remarked.

### Research Gaps in Understanding Wound Healing

Gaps in understanding persist in this area, Moore noted. For instance, it is unclear how B cells adapt in the wound environment. Additionally, researchers do not know whether the B-cell role either in local tissue response or in secreting antibodies informs the systemic response. Moore remarked on her interest in understanding how to connect the local injury response to systemic immunity by linking the B-cell responses at the local and systemic response sites. Furthermore, research that leverages biomaterial models could elucidate patient-specific wound healing, she added. If biomaterials can mimic different wound-healing conditions and microenvironments of vulnerable populations, the contribution of patient variability—including ancestry, age, biological sex, and history of trauma—in wound healing could be interrogated.

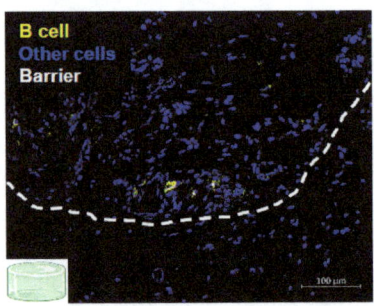
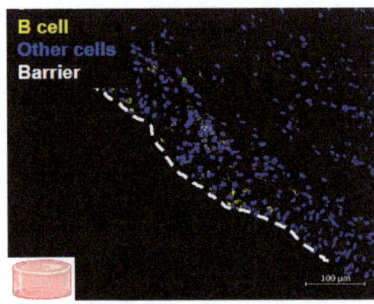
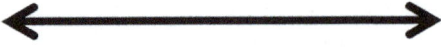

**FIGURE 5-1** Immune response to pro-healing versus pro-fibrotic biomaterials implanted in breast tissue.
SOURCE: Moore presentation, November 2, 2021.

# ENDOGENOUS PRO-RESOLUTION AND PRO-REGENERATIVE MECHANISMS IN PERIODONTAL TISSUE

George Hajishengallis, Thomas W. Evans Centennial Professor in the Department of Basic and Translational Sciences at the University of Pennsylvania, characterized periodontitis as a chronic inflammatory disease that leads to the destruction of tissues that surround and support the teeth—the gingiva, periodontal ligament, and alveolar bone. As periodontitis progresses, loss of attachment to the teeth occurs and bone becomes severely diminished, which can lead to tooth loss. Severe periodontitis is the sixth-most-prevalent inflammatory condition worldwide, affecting 10 percent of the adult population (Kassebaum et al., 2014). Furthermore, periodontitis is associated with increased risk of systemic comorbidities, including cardiovascular disease, Alzheimer's disease, and diabetes (Hajishengallis and Chavakis, 2021). Periodontitis also poses a significant economic burden, costing the United States approximately $154 billion in annual direct and indirect costs (Botelho et al., 2021). Hajishengallis and his team work toward the goal of promoting both resolution of inflammation and tissue regeneration in the periodontal tissue. To this end, they use a combination of in vitro mechanistic models, animal models, and human studies, including a recent phase IIa clinical trial that showed that a complement C3 inhibitor can promote resolution of periodontal inflammation in human patients (Hasturk et al., 2021).

## The Functions of Developmental Endothelial Locus-1

Developmental endothelial locus-1 (DEL-1) is a molecule believed to stimulate endogenous resolution and regenerative pathways, said Hajishengallis. A secreted 52-kilodalton protein, DEL-1 consists of three epidermal growth factor (EGF)-like repeats in the N terminal and two discoidin I–like domains in the C terminal of the molecule (Yuh et al., 2020). The discoidin I–like domains interact with phospholipids, whereas the EGF-like repeats are responsible for interactions with various integrins, transmembrane receptors that bind to the extracellular matrix (Kourtzelis et al., 2019). DEL-1 is expressed primarily by tissue-resident cells, including endothelial cells, neuronal cells, and mesenchymal stem cells (MSC) in the periodontal ligament and bone marrow, and by certain macrophage subsets. Unfortunately, the expression of DEL-1 decreases substantially with aging in both humans and in mice, he noted. DEL-1 was identified as an important molecule with the discovery that it can bind lymphocyte function–associated antigen 1 (LFA-1) on leukocytes such as neutrophils, explained Hajishengallis. DEL-1 blocks the interaction of LFA-1 with the endothelial intercellular adhesion molecule 1, known as ICAM-1 (Choi et al., 2008).

This interaction is important for circulating neutrophils to adhere onto the endothelium and is a prerequisite step for their transmigration, he added.

When DEL-1 is secreted by endothelial cells, it can regulate the recruitment of inflammatory cells into underlying tissues. Hajishengallis and colleagues showed that DEL-1 could confer protection against periodontitis in both mice and nonhuman primates (Eskan et al., 2012; Shin et al., 2015). They extended these observations beyond periodontitis to other disease models by showing that DEL-1 can protect against multiple sclerosis by inhibiting inflammation (Choi et al., 2015). Recently, they demonstrated that DEL-1 is also protective against rheumatoid arthritis (Wang et al., 2021). He emphasized that location influences the functional role of DEL-1. When DEL-1 is expressed by endothelial cells, its job is to regulate neutrophil recruitment. However, when DEL-1 is produced by macrophages, the protein promotes efferocytosis and inflammation resolution because it can serve as a molecular bridge to facilitate the interaction of apoptotic neutrophils with macrophages (Kourtzelis et al., 2019). Specifically, DEL-1 binds phosphatidylserine (PS) on apoptotic cells through its discoidin I–like domains and beta 3 integrin on macrophages through an arginine-glycine-aspartic acid (RGD) motif of the second EGF repeat, thereby promoting the ability of macrophages to engulf apoptotic cells (Kourtzelis et al., 2019). Hajishengallis explained that DEL-1–mediated uptake of apoptotic neutrophils has a function beyond waste disposal. That is, the efferocytic macrophage becomes pro-resolving and begins secreting transforming growth factor (TGF) beta, resolvins, and other factors important for resolving inflammation. This is the mechanism by which DEL-1 promotes inflammation resolution in periodontitis (Kourtzelis et al., 2019).

### Role of Developmental Endothelial Locus-1 in Periodontitis

Researchers have found that DEL-1 can also induce regeneration of bone in periodontitis through an independent mechanism (Yuh et al., 2020). Hajishengallis and his colleagues have used a mouse model in which they induced experimental periodontitis by ligation at the molar teeth, causing accumulation of the biofilm that produces inflammation and subsequently results in alveolar bone loss. At day 10 the ligature was removed, facilitating transition to the resolution phase. Wild-type mice regenerated bone during the resolution phase, whereas the DEL-1–deficient mice did not (Yuh et al., 2020). When DEL-1 knockout mice received a local administration of recombinant DEL-1, the ability to regenerate bone was restored. Surprisingly, the effect of bone regeneration was restored even with the local administration of a segment of DEL-1 consisting of only EGF-like repeats, suggesting that the mechanism depends on EGF-like repeats and does not require the discoidin I–like domains, Hajishengallis said.

A key implication of these data is that the mechanism by which DEL-1 regenerates bone is independent of its ability to promote efferocytosis and resolution, stated Hajishengallis. Inflammation resolution is also important for bone regeneration, but it is significant that DEL-1 carries out these two functions independently, he emphasized. The entire DEL-1 molecule is required for efferocytosis, with one part binding to the macrophages and the other part binding to the apoptotic neutrophils (Kourtzelis et al., 2019). However, the EGF-like repeats alone were sufficient for bone regeneration (Yuh et al., 2020). Hajishengallis and his team also found that the RGD motif in the second EGF-like repeat is critical for bone regeneration. Using a transgenic mouse model with a mutation in the RGD motif of DEL-1 that substituted glutamic acid for aspartic acid, they demonstrated that the mice were unable to regenerate bone during the resolution of periodontitis without this vital domain (Yuh et al., 2020).

In vitro mechanistic studies were used to confirm the in vivo findings, said Hajishengallis. Experiments using a culture model with calvarial osteoblastic cells confirmed that the RGD motif and EGF repeats mediate the ability of DEL-1 to induce osteogenic differentiation and calcified nodule formation (Yuh et al., 2020). Researchers used MC3T3-E1 osteoblastic progenitor cells to dissect the pathway by which DEL-1 promotes osteogenic differentiation. The pathway involves the binding of DEL-1 to the beta 3 integrin, which activates the focal adhesion kinase (FAK); downstream, this prompts both activation of the extracellular signal-regulated protein kinase, known as ERK1/2, and phosphorylation of runt-related transcription factor 2 (RUNX2) (Yuh et al., 2020). RUNX2 is a master regulator of osteogenesis, and DEL-1 promotes osteogenesis by activating RUNX2, noted Hajishengallis. Furthermore, DEL-1 activation of FAK has been shown to activate activate Akt, a group of kinases involved in many cellular functions. Although it is not yet known what the Akt signaling pathway leads to in this context, Hajishengallis suggested that it likely promotes survival of the generated osteoblasts.

## Relationship between Age, Developmental Endothelial Locus-1 Levels, and Bone Regeneration

Young mice were able to regenerate bone during the resolution phase in this model of periodontitis, but old mice failed to do so, highlighted Hajishengallis. Since DEL-1 levels diminish in old age, he and his colleagues are actively researching a hypothesis that the inability of old mice to regenerate bone is, at least in part, due to diminished DEL-1 levels. Given that DEL-1 is expressed in the MSC niche of the periodontal ligament, they believe that the aging-related DEL-1 deficiency contributes to stem cell niche dysfunction in the periodontal ligament, he explained. This in turn may contribute to defective osteogenesis and compromise periodontal tissue repair in old age. Therefore, he and his team are working to reverse the effects of aging in, or rejuvenate, the MSC niche and promote bone regeneration in old age using two DEL-1–based strategies. The first approach involves exogenous administration of recombinant DEL-1. The second approach involves stimulation of endogenous DEL-1 expression in old age, and thus far researchers have identified two molecules that stimulate this expression. Dehydroepiandrosterone (DHEA), a steroid hormone, promotes the production of DEL-1 at both the mRNA and the protein levels (Ziogas et al., 2020). DHEA levels decrease with age in both men and women, and declining DEL-1 levels are possibly associated with declining DHEA levels, Hajishengallis speculated. He added that there is already a need to supplement DHEA levels in older adults because these levels decrease with age and that doing so may also stimulate DEL-1 expression. The other molecule identified as having the ability to stimulate DEL-1 expression is erythromycin, an antibiotic (Maekawa et al., 2020). Hajishengallis, his research team, and their collaborators in Japan are currently experimenting with modified erythromycin that does not have antibiotic activity, yet maintains the ability to upregulate DEL-1.

## DISCUSSION

### Role of Local Environment in Molecular Response

Becker asked Hajishengallis to expand upon the role of the local environment in how a signal is acted upon, whether this can be manipulated, and, if so, how specific the targeting for these types of proteins or factors should be. Hajishengallis responded that studies with DEL-1 demonstrated that location matters. When the same molecule is expressed in a different part of the tissue, it mediates a different function. For example, when DEL-1 was overexpressed in endothelial cells, its only function in blocking inflammation was inhibition of neutrophil recruitment (Kourtzelis et al., 2019). Overexpression of DEL-1 in macrophages does not affect the recruitment of inflammatory cells and instead promotes efferocytosis and inflammation resolution. The experimental technique of quantitative PCR, or qPCR, can be used to determine the increase or decrease of certain molecules in homogenized tissue. However, the utility of these data is limited due to the significance of the location—in terms of the cell type or part of the tissue—where the protein is expressed, Hajishengallis elaborated. The cell type by which DEL-1 mediates bone regeneration is unknown, although the MSCs in the periodontal ligament are likely responsible because they express DEL-1, he acknowledged. Should this be proven, it would signify that DEL-1 expressed in the MSC niche promotes differentiation of MSCs into osteoblast progenitors that then become osteoblasts. Manipulating this function in older adults would involve local, exogenous administration, suggested Hajishengallis. While this means the product could not be targeted to specific cells, the method has worked in mice. Endogenous production of DEL-1 might also be stimulated by other drugs, he added.

## Manipulation of the Local Environment in Tissue Regeneration

A participant asked whether there is a difference in the response of satellite cells to toxins versus exercise-induced muscle damage. Blau replied that both types of damage yield a MuSC response and wave of inflammation and that PGE2 and the series of effects she outlined earlier—including fibroblasts, fibroadipocytes, and the activation of stem cells—are part of that wave. She stated that toxins and exercise can both cause damage that induces potent responses, but to her knowledge, a side-by-side comparison between the two has not been performed.

Given that the local environment affects stem cells, Becker asked how components of the environments can be manipulated to support tissue regeneration. Blau answered that more study is needed on how the niche is affected, what the components of the niches are, and how they change through perturbations. Characterizing the endogenous niche factor PGE2 led to the unexpected discovery of its profound biological effects, she commented. They learned that PGE2 is required for stem cell function, regeneration, and maintenance of muscle fibers, and that it can overcome the wasting that occurs with aging. Inflammation is often regarded as having a negative effect—and chronic inflammation can indeed cause tissue disruption—however, transient inflammation can be beneficial, said Blau. By interrogating a niche factor, the inflammatory metabolite PGE2, she and her colleagues found that restoring it to youthful levels carries benefit. Therefore, manipulating normal signals and studying immune factors can lead to enlisting them in a positive way, she said.

Hajishengallis remarked that most of the cell types he has studied using the DEL-1 model show severely diminished DEL-1 expression. For example, the MSCs in bone marrow express much lower levels of DEL-1 in old age. Stimulating endogenous DEL-1 expression or administering it exogenously is likely to rejuvenate MSCs. This is expected to not only affect the ability of MSCs to differentiate into osteoblasts and other lineages but also have a more general effect on the immune system. He noted that the MSC niche is important for hematopoietic stem cells. As people age, senescence can be limited through targeted reversal of these processes, said Hajishengallis. Capitalizing on endogenous mechanisms, such as the effect of DEL-1 in bone regeneration and of PGE2 in muscle regeneration, can promote healing even as people reach older age.

Moore noted the importance of understanding the difference between injury and homeostasis in the endogenous environment. Areas that merit more research include how the injury environment specifically signals a response to damage, how aging alters the microenvironment of injury, and how to interrogate the signals present or absent at that injury site. For instance, the pro-healing material she has studied delivers extracellular matrix that has been stripped of cells to stimulate a type 2 immune response at the wound site. Researchers are working to understand whether that can be leveraged to promote healing in older individuals by manipulating the endogenous injury site to recreate the injury microenvironments present in a younger person, she elaborated.

## Biomaterials and the Mechanisms of Immune Response

Becker asked Moore about the nature of the biomaterials used in her mouse model. Moore replied that an acellular hydrogel-like mesh network naturally derived from porcine cells was used as the pro-healing material. In contrast, a synthetically derived material called polycaprolactone (PCL) was used for the pro-fibrotic material. Both of these have commercial approval, are used in patients, and are known to guide the immune system toward fibrosis or toward healing. Becker inquired further about the properties of these biomaterials that skew the immune response in wound healing. Moore said that these biomaterials were created specifically for their function. Now that these materials have established wider clinical use, researchers are exploring the mechanisms behind the response, she added. For instance, the naturally derived class of materials is biologically recognizable. Extracellular matrix proteins are largely conserved, and it is possible that the body can recognize and clear them after injury by inducing a type 2 immune response, said Moore. She and her colleagues are working to understand which antigens are responsible for various responses by conducting sequencing work and VDJ (variable, diversity, joining) assessment. Synthetically derived materials are not biologically active, yet they induce either protein denaturation or various DAMPs and PAMPs (damage-associated molecular patterns and pathogen-associated molecular patterns) that can accelerate chronic inflammation and promote a type 17 response that propagates in fibrosis, she continued. Moore remarked that these mechanisms are currently supported by evidence and that she and her team are researching others.

## Cell Involvement and Timing in Pro-Healing Biomaterial

A participant asked whether any other healing cells are attracted to the pro-healing gel in the wound microenvironment, given that Moore and her team have been able to target a specific immune cell, the B cell.

Moore replied that the immunology community is collectively working to map what happens with every known type of immune cell and characterize the interactions between them. Researchers have profiled macrophages, dendritic cells, and T helper (Th) cells, and CD8T cells may be the "last frontier" after the B-cell work that has been conducted, she remarked (Rieckmann et al., 2019; Walsh et al., 2015). Beyond profiling individual cell types, understanding the intracellular communications between different types of immune cells that are recruited to these sites is an area of interest. The observations from studying B cells will complement what is already known about Th2 cells in pro-healing environments and about Th17 cells in pro-fibrotic environments.

Becker asked whether timing is important in manipulating and modulating the immune system and whether a signal can become detrimental later in the timeline. Moore responded that timing is subjective and dependent on each patient, such that a patient-centric approach may be necessary to optimize therapeutics. In the context of an inflammatory cascade, B cells displayed a toggling effect dependent on timing of recruitment. Specifically, recruiting B cells earlier in the healing timeframe had a more pro-regenerative effect. When recruitment to the injury site took place later, B cells were more likely to be antigen-experienced, and thus promote fibrosis. More profiling would help to understand the differences responsible for that toggling effect and to determine why recruiting mature B cells later did not occur to the same extent with the pro-healing material, Moore added. Timing is important with all immunological cascades, specifically with regard to wound healing, she stated. Research on timing can inform identification of general hallmarks, which in turn could be applied to each patient to understand their individual response. For instance, if a patient has B cells that are recruited later, that could indicate a fibrotic response, and this response could be mapped, she elaborated.

## Silicone Implants and B-Cell Response

Blau remarked that the area of breast implants warrants attention because women who have their breasts removed due to cancer do not have adequate options with silicone implants. Blau asked Moore whether she is pursuing the identification of materials that promote better regrowth of tissue. Moore replied that she and her colleagues have been profiling a host of cells in addition to B cells. Other labs have profiled the response of gamma-delta T cells, other T cells, and fibroblasts to silicone breast implants. She highlighted research efforts by the Elisseeff Lab and the Doloff Lab for Immunoengineering and Regenerative Medicine at Johns Hopkins University in profiling immune cell responses (Chung et al., 2020). Interestingly, B-cell dysfunction in the presence of synthetically implanted biomaterials has tenuous connections with autoimmunity development; some people with silicone breast implants have a higher likelihood of developing autoimmune disorders or B-cell–related cancers, Moore explained. Her team is working to understand the role of B cells at that site and why they may be important despite their relatively small population size in comparison to other immune cells. Moore expressed her interest in pursuing the connection between implants and autoimmunity, the relationship between implants and the continuing response to trauma or injury, the effect of repetitive trauma on both the B-cell and general immune response, and how B cells are taught tolerance through injury.

Hajishengallis inquired whether the phenotype of the recruited B cells has been analyzed, and if so, whether they are regulatory B cells (Breg) that secrete interleukin-10 (IL-10). Moore replied that her lab profiled the peritoneum and the spleen to study the systemic response after a muscle injury. B10- or Breg-positive cells were not detected at the injury site. Bregs are housed largely in peritoneal fluid and were detected there, but the difference between the percentage of Bregs before and after injury was not statistically significant. In order to confirm the maturity of B cells on implanted material, Moore and her team used commonly known surface markers, such as CD138. The profiling of those cells is in progress to understand whether class switching is taking place and whether the cells are tolerant. Additionally, her team has studied B1A and B1B cells, which are antigen-immature, continually secrete broad immunoglobulins, but were not detected in the injury site. Ongoing profiling of this class of B cells should reveal how Bregs respond in the peritoneum and in comparison both to B1A and B1B cells and to other parts of the tissue, noted Moore.

### Combining Cellular Therapy Modalities

Becker asked the panelists how immune system modulation can influence transplantation technique in harnessing the immune system to make exogenous replacement therapies more effective. Hajishengallis responded that apoptosis appears to be a major mechanism by which transplanted MSCs promote resolution of inflammation and protection against autoimmune diseases (Galleu et al., 2017). Apoptotic MSCs are taken up by macrophages, and the efferocytic macrophages are reprogrammed to become pro-resolving macrophages. For this mechanism to be effective in older adults, molecules such as DEL-1 or other molecular bridges must be present, he added. Therefore, transplantation of MSCs to treat autoimmune disease may garner different results in younger people than in older people, and it may not be sufficient to achieve benefit in the older population. Stimulating the endogenous expression of DEL-1 and similar molecules, such as milk fat globule-EGF factor 8 protein (MFGE8), or supplying it exogenously could potentially be combined with cell transplantation to enhance therapeutic effectiveness.

Blau emphasized that combining modalities can be powerful, noting that a process of isolating MuSCs and coinjecting them with PGE2 into injured muscles has resulted in faster, more robust muscle repair associated with increases in muscle strength. Moore added that MSCs are particularly immunomodulatory and immune sensitive, and that manipulating the carriers used for MSC injection—perhaps by injecting them in a hydrogel mesh—might promote immune cell recruitment. Opportunities to marry the fields of endogenous immune modulation and exogenous cell replacement therapy include shifting the immunological response to cell therapies and could leverage the benefits of both, Moore suggested. For instance, bodies can respond to cell therapies in undesirable ways, such as with macrophage phagocytosis. If the macrophage function could be manipulated from a phagocytic M1 paradigm to an M2 paradigm, this may foster the body's ability to regenerate tissue and control how the body responds to implanted cells, she explained. Moore underscored her excitement about interdisciplinary approaches that leverage one another.

## Use of Complex versus Simple Models

Given that a variety of experimental models are in use, Becker asked about the pros and cons of conducting this research in a complex system, such as in an animal or in vivo model, versus in a less complex system with an in vitro or organoid approach. Moore replied that she and her team are involved in a suite of research that focuses on an in vitro approach. In vivo studies can yield information about mechanisms involved in a process, but these studies can be overly complicated. In vitro applications allow for the study of cell-to-cell interactions, such as communication between an isolated patient cell and another desired cell type, to understand the "crosstalk" between each cell in terms of soluble, juxtacrine, paracrine, and other forms of signaling. Biomaterial models provide opportunities to make the most of what both in vivo and in vitro systems have to offer, said Moore.

Hajishengallis commented that his lab focuses on preclinical models and in vitro models that can facilitate understanding mechanisms and signaling that cannot be carried out with in vivo models. Human studies are also used to validate findings from preclinical models. These may be correlative studies to confirm relevance or human trials, such as the phase II clinical trial of a drug that he and his team developed (Hasturk et al., 2021). He expressed hope that DEL-1 will eventually be tested in humans, a step toward the ultimate goal of curing patients. Blau remarked that no treatments for aging, sarcopenia, and loss of muscle mass are currently approved, and she also hopes her mouse studies will translate to clinical trials to improve people's quality of life.

# 6

# Modulating the Host Immune System to Create a Pro-Regenerative Environment

**Key Points Highlighted by Individual Speakers**

- Fundamental aging processes are linked, so interventions that target one pathway tend to affect the rest. (Kirkland)
- Senolytic agents are unique because they target senescent cells, not a single molecule or pathway like more traditional one-drug, one-target, one-disease approaches. They can delay, prevent, or alleviate senescence and age-related conditions and diseases. (Kirkland)
- The combination of senolytics and anti-fibrotic agents can have a synergistic pro-healing effect. (Kirkland)
- Regenerative immunology marries the fields of regenerative medicine, immunology, and biomaterial design to develop novel engineered therapies to promote endogenous tissue regeneration. (Elisseeff)
- The future of immunotherapies will likely include combination therapies to promote productive tissue regeneration and inhibit fibrotic responses. (Elisseeff)
- Resolving inflammation stimulates regeneration via pro-resolving mediators, which are distinct from anti-inflammatory compounds that may interfere with the beneficial effects of inflammation. (Serhan)
- Optimal timing for treatment intervention differs across organs and tissues and needs to be customized. (Serhan)

The fourth session of the workshop focused on efforts to modulate the host immune system to create a pro-regenerative environment. The session's objectives were to (1) discuss the goal of host immune modulation and consider what the correct molecular targets are for creating a pro-regenerative environment and (2) examine recent advances of the role of innate and adaptive immunity in cell engraftment and endogenous tissue regeneration, and approaches for immunomodulation of the structure and function of stem cell niches for goals of tissue regeneration. The session was moderated by Candace Kerr, program officer of the Stem Cell Program of the Aging Physiology Branch at the National Institute on Aging.

## CELLULAR SENESCENCE, SENOLYTICS, AND ORGAN REGENERATION AND TRANSPLANTATION

James Kirkland, director of the Robert and Arlene Kogod Center on Aging and Noaber Foundation Professor of Aging Research at the Mayo Clinic, discussed fundamental aging processes and their effects on issues related to organ regeneration and transplantation.

### Unitary Theory of Fundamental Aging Mechanisms

Fundamental aging processes begin at the time of conception, Kirkland stated. These processes, which are largely conserved across vertebrate species, can be classified into between four and 13 different categories or "pillars" of aging. Increasing evidence that these processes are interlinked, such that targeting one tends to affect the rest, underpins the unitary theory of fundamental aging processes (see Box 6-1), he explained. In addition, the geroscience hypothesis put forth by Gordon Lithgow holds that interventions modifying aging biology can slow its progression, thereby delaying or preventing the onset of multiple diseases and disorders (Sierra et al., 2021). Moreover, fundamental aging processes may be root-cause contributors to the majority of conditions that cause most morbidity, mortality, and health expenditures (see Box 6-1). In addition to aging phenotypes and geriatric syndromes (e.g., sarcopenia, frailty), these conditions include major chronic diseases—many of which still lack effective treatments—as well as decreased ability to withstand an infection, respond to a vaccine, or to recover after chemotherapy. Importantly, interventions that target any one of these fundamental aging processes will tend to affect all the others, Kirkland emphasized.

> **BOX 6-1**
> **Fundamental Aging Mechanisms and Phenotypes**
>
> Fundamental aging mechanisms:
> - Inflammation (chronic, low grade, sterile), fibrosis
> - Macromolecular and/or organelle dysfunction (e.g., DNA, protein aggregates, autophagy, advanced glycation end products, lipotoxicity, mitochondrial dysfunction)
> - Stem cell and progenitor dysfunction
> - Cellular senescence
>
> Phenotypes of aging:
> - Geriatric syndromes: sarcopenia, frailty, immobility, mild cognitive impairment
> - Chronic diseases: dementias, cancers, atherosclerosis, diabetes, osteoporosis, osteoarthritis, renal dysfunction, blindness, chronic lung disease
> - Decreased resilience: infections, delirium, delayed wound healing, slow rehabilitation, chemotherapy toxicity, ICU care
>
> SOURCES: Kirkland presentation, November 3, 2021; adapted from Palmer et al., 2019, under the Creative Commons license (http://creativecommons.org/licenses/by/4.0/).

### Transient, Beneficial versus Persistent, Deleterious Senescent Cells

Senescent cells accumulate not only with aging, but also at sites of age-related diseases, diseases in younger individuals, and multiple acute and chronic diseases, Kirkland explained. Senescent cells can be sorted into two groups: those that are acutely generated and beneficial versus those that are persistent and deleterious, he described. Newly formed senescent cells have lost the ability to divide but remain alive and can have myriad beneficial functions that include secreting a range of cytokines, chemokines, proteases, growth factors, noncoding nucleotides, and bioactive lipids. Furthermore, acutely generated senescent cells defend against cancer development and infection and support wound healing and tissue remodeling. Even in seemingly unrelated processes like parturition, senescent cells accumulate in the placenta and produce factors that drive the neonate through the birth canal. Since many physiological functions depend on the acute generation of transient senescent cells, Kirkland cautioned against interfering with the capacity of such cells to become senescent, which could lead to cancer development or failed wound healing. Although many or most senescent cells can produce senescent-associated secretory phenotype (SASP) factors, approximately 30–70 percent of persistent senescent cells may have a tissue-destructive, pro-apoptotic SASP, which appears to contribute to a host of deleterious effects and accentuate the other pillars of aging (Tripathi et al.,

2021). For example, persistent, SASP-expressing, pro-apoptotic senescent cells can result in (1) increased inflammation, fibrosis, and stem and progenitor cell dysfunction; (2) decreased levels of proteins such as nicotinamide adenine dinucleotide and α-Klotho; (3) elevated CD38 and mammalian target of rapamycin (mTOR); (4) increased likelihood of cancers and chronic disease; and (5) the spread of senescence.

### Effects of Transplanting Senescent Cells

Murine models have been used to study the effects of transplanted senescent cells. For instance, transplanting relatively small numbers of senescent cells into a middle-aged mouse can cause physical dysfunction and result in premature death, Kirkland described (Xu et al., 2018). Transplanting 1 million senescent cells—such that scarcely one in 10,000 cells in the mouse is a transplanted senescent cell—is sufficient to drive frailty in those mice (Xu et al., 2018). The mice exhibit decreased strength, as shown by reduced hanging endurance and ability to run on a treadmill, and they tend to die early after a lag period. Mice with transplanted senescent cells tend to die prematurely due to all typical age-related diseases, not any specific disease, Kirkland highlighted. These findings support a causal link between senescent cells and multimorbidity, since adding a small number of senescent cells can accelerate age-related health problems and death from all causes (Xu et al., 2018).

Evidence also indicates that transplanted senescent cells can spread senescence to non-senescent host cells in both paracrine and endocrine manners, said Kirkland. By labeling senescent cells that were transplanted into a middle-aged mouse, researchers determined whether observed senescent cells originated from the transplanted senescent cells or if the recipients' own cells became senescent (Xu et al., 2018). Remarkably, if senescent cells are transplanted into the peritoneum, the recipients' cells in their arms and legs start becoming senescent, he said. The immune system normally removes senescent cells; however, these results suggest that, above a threshold burden, new senescent cells can be formed due to the spread of senescence at a rate that exceeds the ability of the immune system to clear them, Kirkland posited. When that threshold is surpassed, a range of deleterious effects may result. Experimental evidence from mouse studies further supports this postulated threshold phenomenon, he added. As previously described, approximately 1 million transplanted senescent cells are sufficient to cause dysfunction in a middle-aged mouse receiving a normal diet, but a transplant of only 500,000 cells has no injurious effect. Whereas, in old mice or middle-aged mice on a high-fat diet, a transplant of 500,000 cells can cause the recipient mouse to become frail and die prematurely (Xu et al., 2018). The outcome indicates that these mice are already closer to the senescent-cell threshold burden due to the greater number of preexisting senescent cells in old or obese animals.

In another mouse study, transplantation of cardiac allografts from old donors also induced cellular senescence in young recipient organs, Kirkland observed. By comparing the effects of transplanting hearts from old mice into young mice versus from young mice into other young mice, researchers found that senescent cells from the hearts of the old mice spread senescence to other organs of the young mice (Iske et al., 2020). This occurs in much the same way as transplanting senescent cells into young mice, Kirkland commented. Furthermore, the 30–70 percent of senescent cells that have a pro-apoptotic, tissue-damaging SASP can secrete noncoding nucleotides, including mitochondrial DNA. Iske and colleagues showed that mitochondrial DNA produced by senescent cells in the hearts from the old mice activates dendritic cells in draining lymph nodes and substantially accelerates graft-versus-host disease (Iske et al., 2020). Kirkland noted that this effect is appreciated by transplant surgeons who are reluctant to transplant organs from old donors to young recipients, contributing to large numbers of nonutilized organs from consenting donors each year.

### Hypothesis-Driven Senolytic Drug Development

For the past two decades, a new avenue of research has emphasized hypothesis-driven senolytic drug development, said Kirkland. In a seminal publication in 2004, Ned Sharpless and his colleagues found that caloric restriction, which increases healthspan, could reduce senescent cell accumulation as well as delay frailty and the onset of age-related diseases (Krishnamurthy et al., 2004). This work gave rise to questions about possible causal effects of eliminating senescent cells on morbidity and laid the groundwork for the lengthy process of developing drugs that would selectively target those senescent cells.

Given that the 30–70 percent of senescent cells with a tissue-destructive SASP survive despite killing the other cells around them, Kirkland and his team asked whether such senescent cells may have defenses against their own pro-apoptotic signaling. Through bioinformatics, an entire series of interlinked pathways emerged, forming a network termed the senescent cell anti-apoptotic pathway (SCAP) network. The networked anti-apoptotic regulator pathways confer resistance to apoptosis in senescent cells. Efforts to identify agents that target nodes in the network or along those pathways have yielded approximately 40–50 candidate drugs, Kirkland said. In particular, agents with short elimination half-lives are sought in order to kill or remove senescent cells in an intermittent "hit-and-run" fashion, given that it takes one to six weeks for new senescent cells to form in cell culture, he added. Since senolytic drugs target senescent cells rather than a single molecule or pathway, the paradigm is analogous to developing antibiotics that could treat multiple types of infection, in contrast to the traditional one-drug, one-molecular-target, one-disease strategy, Kirkland highlighted.

Research into the mechanism of action of the senolytic agents has revealed that different types of senescent cells depend on different elements of the SCAP network for their survival, Kirkland stated. For instance, dasatinib is a Src kinase inhibitor that is senolytic for human fat cell progenitors but not for endothelial cells because human senescent fat cell progenitors rely on ephrin-dependent survival pathways to defend themselves against their own SASP. In contrast, endothelial-cell defense mechanisms depend more heavily on B-cell lymphoma 2 family members, p21-related pathways, and heat shock protein 90, so quercetin, a flavonoid, was effective against senescent human umbilical vein endothelial cells (HUVECs). Since dasatinib did not kill senescent HUVECs and quercetin did not kill senescent pre-adipocytes, a combination of the two agents was investigated in mice and was able to eliminate a broader range of senescent cell types than either agent could alone (Zhu et al., 2015). Furthermore, a comparison of transplanted luciferase-expressing senescent cells versus non-senescent cells showed that the 30–70 percent of senescent cells with a pro-apoptotic, tissue-damaging SASP were eliminated by allowing them to "commit suicide" based on their own SASP, Kirkland explained (Xu et al., 2018).

A series of other senolytics has been developed using these approaches and others, and the senolytics can delay, prevent, or alleviate more than 60 conditions in mice, Kirkland said. Although the translation of drugs from mouse to human is not straightforward, senolytics alleviated frailty when given to animals with transplanted senescent cells (Xu et al., 2018). In heart-transplanted animals, senolytics were associated with reduced rejection rates (Iske et al., 2020). Moreover, promising evidence suggests that treating the donor, the recipient, or even the heart itself with senolytics can potentially reduce rejection and death in mice, offering the potential to utilize greater numbers of older donor organs, remarked Kirkland.

However, it is not yet clear that the effects of senolytics in mice will safely translate to humans, noted Kirkland. To explore the safety and efficacy of these agents in humans, clinical trials of senolytics have already been initiated.[1] Publications about the first-in-human clinical trials of senolytics have found that the agents can clear senescent cells effectively from human adipose tissue, for example (Hickson et al., 2019). Blood measures of senescence based on composite scores indicate that senolytic agents can reduce senescent cells through intermittent treatment. Within the Translational Geroscience Network, 15 clinical trials are underway to examine the effects of different senolytics on conditions such as frailty, Alzheimer's disease,

---

[1] ClinicalTrials.gov identifier: NCT02848131.

diabetes-related kidney disease, idiopathic pulmonary fibrosis, osteoporosis, and osteoarthritis. One study is investigating the effect of senolytics after bone marrow transplantation in an attempt to delay the accelerated aging-like state that can develop three to five years after the transplant. Another study in childhood cancer survivors is using senolytics to attempt to reduce the incidence of the associated accelerated aging-like state. Three trials are also underway for coronavirus in inpatients, outpatients, and nursing home residents. A lot of work remains to be done to ensure safe translation of senolytic therapeutics to humans, Kirkland emphasized.

## MAPPING THE IMMUNE AND TISSUE ENVIRONMENT IN HEALING AND NON-HEALING WOUNDS

Jennifer Elisseeff, Morton Goldberg Professor of Ophthalmology and Biomedical Engineering and director of the Translational Tissue Engineering Center at Johns Hopkins University, shared efforts to map the immune and tissue environment in healing and non-healing wounds.

Tissue and organ loss remains a global issue, said Elisseeff. Although transplantation can provide functional tissues for those suffering from tissue and organ loss, the major challenges of immune rejection and tolerance persist. Similarly, synthetic implants (e.g., cartilage, breast, and others) are associated with challenges because they do not recapitulate all tissue functions. These two fields and their limitations led to the development of tissue engineering, which aims to provide new healthy tissue by taking a biomaterial scaffold that serves as a three-dimensional framework for components like stem cells and where specified biological signals can promote tissue development. Unfortunately, clinical translation of tissue engineering discoveries has been slow, Elisseeff remarked.

### Rebuilding Cartilage in Patients

In the early stages of tissue engineering research, Elisseeff and colleagues targeted cartilage tissue that lines the surface of joints because, when damaged, cartilage tissue cannot heal well. Elisseeff and colleagues began by designing materials to stimulate stem cell development and recapitulate elements of normal developmental biology to build replacement cartilage tissue, she explained. This work led to the development of therapies that combined synthetic and biological materials and could be incorporated with surgical practice to mobilize endogenous cells to promote tissue repair (Sharma et al., 2013; Wang et al., 2007). After 12 months, the surgical microfracture process leads to fibrocartilage that degrades over time;

however, tissue volume and quality can be maintained with a biomaterial scaffold (Sharma et al., 2013).

Clinical translation informed a new research direction when it became clear that this process did not recapitulate the elements of classical tissue engineering; instead, the treatment redirected the wound-healing process, Elisseeff said. Another clinical trial further demonstrated that there is a tissue-specific immune response associated with biomaterial implants (Hillel et al., 2011). Different types of immune cells and—unexpectedly—T cells were observed depending on which type of tissue was adjacent to the implant, she noted. Based on this discovery, their research focus shifted from classical tissue engineering to focus on the immune system as a key regulator of tissue regeneration and the biomaterial response. The use of biomaterials facilitated the development of models to study different tissue environments and how they mobilize the immune system, she added.

## Regenerative Immunology

Elisseeff explained that the concept of regenerative immunology marries the fields of regenerative medicine, immunology, and tissue engineering (see Figure 6-1). As the first responder to an injury, the immune system sets the stage for subsequent healing processes. Although cells such as macrophages have long been recognized for their role in tissue repair, cells of the adaptive immune system, such as T cells, had not previously been considered as having a critical role. To inform efforts to engineer immunotherapies, Elisseeff and colleagues began mapping these immune responses and investigating how they influence downstream processes such as vascularization, tissue development, and mobilization of different immune cell types. The immune system is therapeutically accessible, making it a prime target for regenerative medicine, she noted.

## Mapping the Natural Immune Response after Tissue Injury

A first step in developing immunotherapies to promote healing is to map the natural immune response after a tissue injury in a healing wound versus a non-healing wound characterized by fibrosis and inflammation, said Elisseeff. Muscle tissue is an example of a healing wound environment, and cartilage is a prototype of a non-healing wound, with biomaterials also modulating the immune environment.

### *Biomaterials Change the Immune Response*

To examine the ability of biomaterials to modulate the immune response, Elisseeff and her team examined a pro-regenerative biological scaffold in a

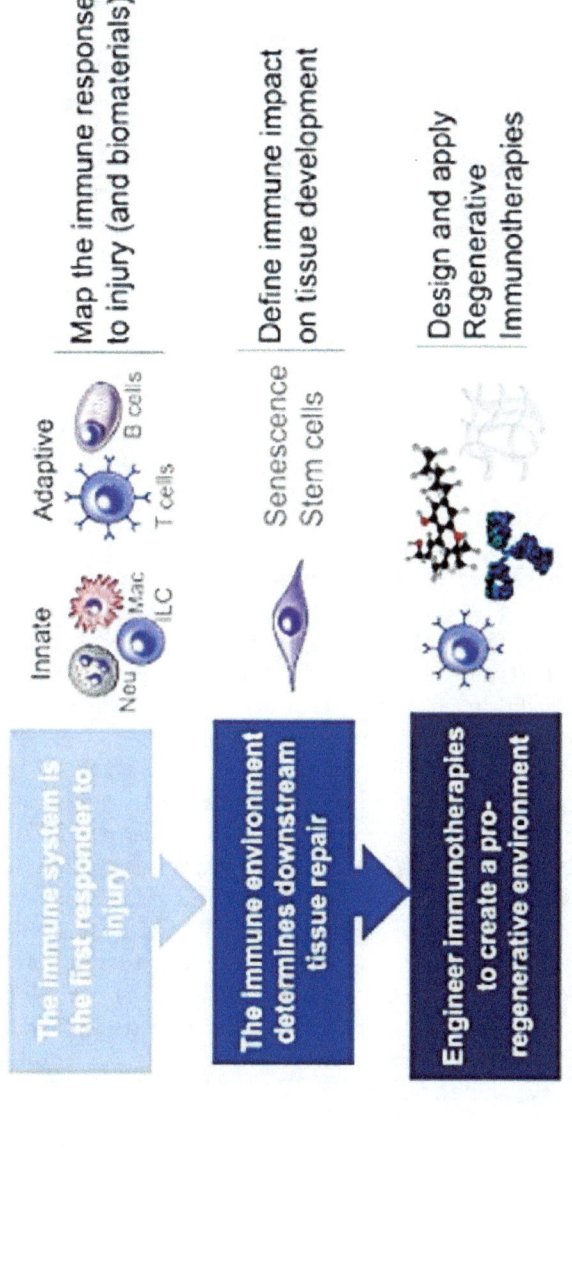

**FIGURE 6-1** Foundations of regenerative immunology.
SOURCE: Elisseeff presentation, November 3, 2021.

muscle wound and found that the biological scaffold stimulates interleukin 4 (IL-4) production by CD4 T cells and others as well as induces macrophage behavior to a pro-regenerative phenotype (Sadtler et al., 2016). Moreover, changes in both local and distal draining lymph nodes demonstrate how local wounds and implants can have systemic implications and, conversely, how the systemic state of the organism can influence a local wound's environment, Elisseeff said. Some differences in the development of repair versus fibrosis depend exclusively on T cells, she added. If an animal without T cells is repopulated with healthy T cells, effective muscle repair can occur. However, if the animal receives T cells deficient in the mTOR complex 2, T helper 2 (Th2) cell differentiation cannot happen, leading to fibrosis and adipogenesis at the injury site (Sadtler et al., 2016).

### Biomaterials-Directed Regenerative Immunology

In contrast to biologically derived biomaterials, synthetic materials are characterized by foreign-body-responsive fibrosis (Chung et al., 2020). For example, fibrosis and collagen are evident with clinical implants of a polyester-based scaffold, Elisseeff described. Whereas the biological scaffold stimulates IL-4, the synthetic material induces production of interleukin 17 (IL-17) by innate lymphocytes, gamma-delta T cells, and T helper 17 (Th17) cells (Chung et al., 2020). However, eliminating IL-17 with a neutralizing antibody can reduce that fibrosis, she noted. This finding is further supported with clinical data. In implants taken from patients and tested for the same markers, the production of elevated IL-17 by CD4 T cells and gamma-delta T cells exceeds the IL-4 interferon gamma production by these T cells around the clinical implants (Chung et al., 2020). The dichotomy of these biomaterial-specific immune responses can be thought of as a balance, Elisseeff described. The biomaterial can influence the environment toward a type 2 IL-4 response, with Th2 and eosinophils playing a major role and providing a healing environment, or the biomaterial can modulate toward a more fibrotic environment in which these cell types are secreting IL-17. This balance can be manipulated slightly by agents that are known to stimulate a type 2 response (e.g., *Schistosoma* soluble egg antigen) or inhibit IL-17, she added.

### Regenerative Immunology and Big Data

Elisseeff and her colleagues are now integrating big data techniques, such as single-cell RNA sequencing, with the biomaterial models to create a large database of single-cell sequencing results from different biomaterial environments. To explore the communication modalities in the healthy versus fibrotic environments, researchers developed a program to examine transcription factor activation in single-cell datasets and construct intercellular signaling networks, which can be grouped into modules (Cherry et al., 2021). Of particular interest is the communication among signaling modules that arise from the analysis, including an immune module, a fibroblast module, and a tissue module. Although some transcription factors and receptor combinations overlap in the different biomaterial and immune environments, others are unique. Elisseeff and her team are also using transfer learning algorithms to identify rare cell types, such as senescent cells, and can learn how the cells participate in immune–stromal communication.

### Immunological Impact of Senescence

In non-healing cartilage wounds, the clearance of senescent cells reduces inflammation and improves tissue repair, Elisseeff commented. Senescent cells can be found in a non-healing cartilage wound characterized by inflammation and arthritis. Clearing senescent cells after injury can promote tissue repair simply by removing inhibitory factors without requiring additional growth factors or stem cells. However, senescent cells are immunologically active and impact multiple immune cell types, she noted. For example, the balance between IL-4 and IL-17 is particularly important for T cells, and the SASP of senescent cells at the injury site includes molecules known to influence them toward the less desirable Th17 pathway.

Further demonstrating this phenomenon, artificially induced senescent fibroblasts that were cultured with naïve T cells in the presence of TGF-beta induced a significant increase in IL-17 (Faust et al., 2020). Conversely, when T cells are guided toward the Th17 phenotype and cultured next to healthy fibroblasts, there is an increase in senescence markers. This phenomenon is referred to as "immunologically induced senescence." In fact, a senescent cell may be considered an immune cell, with both IL-17 and senescent factors playing a role in a positive feed-forward loop, Elisseeff posited. In vivo experiments also provide evidence for immunologically induced senescence. Specifically, components such as gamma-delta T cells can increase IL-17 in the joint, and the lymph node exhibits associated changes. When senescent cells are removed, the IL-17 signature in the joint and lymph node decreases (Faust et al., 2020). In the context of the foreign body response, these findings present new therapeutic targets—namely, senescent cells and the immune factors that are capable of inducing senescence, such as IL-17, Elisseeff emphasized.

### Aging Changes Immune Response to Injury

Aging alters wound repair and regeneration, Elisseeff said, noting that their procedure for local senolysis in the joint was not effective in older animals, who required a combination of local and systemic senolysis (Faust et al., 2020). In the context of muscle injury, IL-4 decreases significantly with aging, while IL-17 increases, in part due to a reduction in Th2 cells and eosinophils. Moreover, older animals have more Th17 and gamma-delta T cells in addition to more CD8 cells, which are pro-inflammatory. Upon investigation, single-cell network and intercellular communication analysis exposed a major disruption in the signaling between the fibroblast module and the immune and antigen-presenting modules in older animals, Elisseeff described. Without injury, old lymph nodes feature fewer naïve T cells than do young lymph nodes. Furthermore, expression profiling of old lymph nodes reveals elevated adipogenesis markers and Th17 differentiation as well as a significant increase of IL-17A and IL-17F at baseline, conditions that the injury exacerbates (Han et al., 2021).

Other markers connected with IL-17 protein interactions increase with injury exclusively in old animals, Elisseeff added. For example, no differences are observed in MMP9[2] between young and old animals without injury (Han et al., 2021). That is, immunological dysfunction exists before injury, and new dysfunction emerges after injury, which "unleashes these signals," she said. Given the baseline immunological dysfunction in old animals, pro-regenerative biomaterial implants can yield poor tissue quality, including fibrosis and adipogenesis, but a combination therapy approach can restore healing in an aged environment, Elisseeff remarked. The combination therapy consisted of pro-regenerative material and an anti–IL-17 neutralizing antibody one week after injury—as treating too early can inhibit immune cell migration and healing. The therapy increased IL-4 produced by T cells, reducing adipogenesis and fibrosis, and recovered some aspects of the repair process, she explained.

### Exploring the Future of Regenerative Immunotherapies

Elisseeff concluded by suggesting key research directions to support future regenerative immunotherapies. Efforts are ongoing to map the immune–stromal response (i.e., the immune response and the range of interconnected cell types that lead to immune changes and regulate tissue repair). This work also introduces new questions of specificity in T-cell memory, senescence–immune connections, and immune sources of variability in tissue repair, she noted. From a clinical perspective, it is well established that genetics can impact an individual's immune response early in life, but later on in life, the immune response is largely dictated by the

---

[2] MMP9 is a subtype of matrix metalloproteinase (MMP). MMPs remodel the extracellular matrix, influencing its composition and cellular processes such as cell growth, movement, and survival (Anderson et al., 2008).

individual's experience of antigens and infections. This factor could be a critical source of variability to consider in regenerative medicine when considering the immune system, she observed.

Many tools are available now to design immunotherapies and, to capitalize on them, research strategies could consider ways to both promote tissue development and remove inhibitory factors that block the tissue repair process, suggested Elisseeff. The immune system also introduces the concept and importance of local and systemic interactions that impact repair processes and therapeutic responses. Finally, interesting connections exist between the wound and the tumor, Elisseeff added. Tumors are often considered to be non-healing wounds, and immunotherapy responsiveness of tumors has been correlated with wound healing signatures. Therefore, leveraging tools of cancer immunology could inform work on wound healing, and wound healing studies can broaden understanding of tumors, she elaborated.

## RESOLUTION OF ACUTE INFLAMMATION STIMULATES TISSUE REGENERATION

Charles Serhan, endowed distinguished scientist and director of the Center for Experimental Therapeutics and Reperfusion Injury at Brigham Women's Hospital and professor of anesthesia at Harvard Medical School, presented evidence that resolving inflammation can stimulate tissue regeneration via novel specialized pro-resolving mediators (SPM), such as the resolvins and microparticles that carry resolvins, lipoxins, and their stable mimetics as payloads.

### Role of Endogenous Control Mechanisms in Resolving Inflammation

The ideal outcome of an acute inflammatory response is complete resolution of inflammation, and endogenous control mechanisms regulate the resolution process (see Figure 6-2). Interrogating pus from mammals and humans has revealed temporal lipid mediators of class switching. An entire family of specialized pro-resolving lipid mediators functions to stimulate resolution and includes the resolvins, the lipoxins, and the protectins, all of which are derived from essential fatty acids (Serhan and Levy, 2018). The two main functions in resolution consist of (1) the cessation of neutrophil infiltration and (2) phagocytosis of apoptotic polymorphonuclear neutrophils (PMNs) by macrophages, known as efferocytosis, as well as clearance of debris, microbes, and fibrin clots. Investigation of these functions of resolution yielded the structural elucidation of each of the pathways. Serhan and his team introduced resolution indices, which are a quantitative

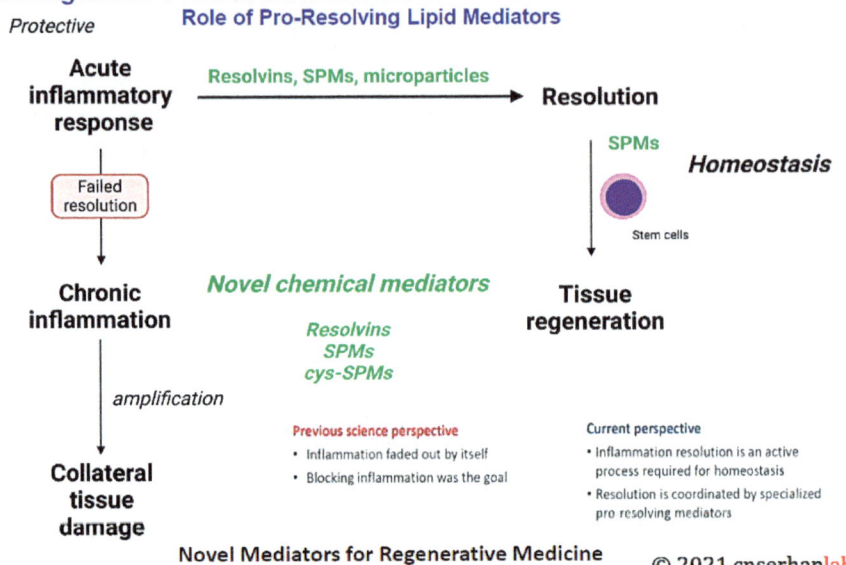

**FIGURE 6-2** Endogenous control mechanisms in resolution of inflammation.
NOTE: SPM = specialized pro-resolving mediator.
SOURCE: Serhan presentation, November 3, 2021.

means of pinpointing where and when the pro-resolving lipid mediators act, he added.

Eventually, it became evident that stimulating resolution is not equivalent to inhibiting inflammation (i.e., pro-resolution is not anti-inflammation) (Serhan et al., 2015). SPMs activate macrophages to uptake apoptotic PMNs, so they are considered immuno-resolvins that stimulate resolution, Serhan explained. Within the range of potencies of the classic pro-inflammatory mediators, the prostaglandins are situated in the middle. Leukotrienes, which are highly potent pro-inflammatory mediators, are in the picomolar to nanomolar range—as are all pro-resolving mediators. As agonists of resolution, the most potent pro-resolving mediators are often referred to as "stop signals" and include lipoxins, resolvins, protectins, and maresins.

### Translational Potential of Specialized Pro-Resolving Mediators

To investigate the action of SPMs in human cells, Serhan and his colleagues used a microfluidic device to simulate human neutrophil swarming and validate "stop" signals. As the first responders to invaders, human neutrophils "swarm like sharks," Serhan said. Adding a pro-resolving mediator can stop the neutrophil swarm, providing direct evidence of the action of SPMs on human neutrophils and suggesting that this type of tool could be used to assess immune status (Reategui et al., 2017). Determining each of the biosynthetic pathways and the complete stereochemistry of each of the bioactive mediators that are formed in these cascades from essential fatty acids has provided an opportunity to identify the pro-resolving functions of SPMs (Serhan, 2014). While the primary function is to shorten the resolution interval, other functions of the SPMs include the following:

- Reducing pro-inflammatory cytokines and their counter-regulation
- Reducing eicosanoid storms
- Enhancing PMN clearance and bacterial killing
- Stimulating phagocytosis of apoptotic PMNs (i.e., efferocytosis)
- Increasing removal of inflammatory debris via lymphatics

SPMs are now commercially available and have a range of confirmed functions in animal disease models, including inflammation resolution, tissue protection, infection control, pain reduction, tissue repair, and wound healing. Importantly, these SPMs are log-orders more potent than nonsteroidal anti-inflammatory agents, Serhan added.

### Novel Mechanism of Action of Specialized Pro-Resolving Mediators

Most SPMs are produced by two cell types—apoptotic PMNs, which are temporally produced during the trafficking of different cells into the inflammatory milieu, and M2 macrophages—in addition to muscle and adipose tissue, Serhan explained. SPMs work through a novel mechanism of action that limits the magnitude and duration of the acute inflammatory response by reducing both eicosanoid (i.e., bioactive lipid mediator) and cytokine storms. They down-regulate prostaglandins, leukotrienes, and chemokines and cytokines and act in a stereo-selective manner on G-protein–coupled receptors to resolve inflammation. In addition to their actions on the innate immune system, the SPMs and resolvins act on components of the adaptive immune system, including T-cell subsets to regulate cytokine production and produce IL-10 and on B cells to regulate antibody production (Chiurchiu et al., 2016; Serhan et al., 2018). Promising research has shown that SPMs can stimulate stem cells, including periodontal stem cells, neural stem cells, mesenchymal stem cells, and muscle stem cells (Cianci et al., 2016; Dort et al., 2021). For instance, SPMs were shown to accelerate wound closure by stimulating periodontal ligament stem cell migration (Markworth et al., 2020).

### Developing Nano Pro-Resolving Medicines

Pro-resolving mediators can be combined with nanoparticles to create nano pro-resolving medicines that mimic endogenous resolution mechanisms, Serhan explained. During the acute inflammatory response, microparticles, which are cell-derived communication vesicles that contain molecular cargo, are released. In the resolution phase of the response, these microvesicles are pro-resolving by carrying intermediates and precursors for resolvins. Serhan and his colleagues mimicked this endogenous resolution phenomenon by creating nanoparticles from human leukocytes and fortifying them with pro-resolving mediators (e.g., resolvin D1) as a therapeutic delivery system (Norling et al., 2011). These enriched nanoparticles have been shown to reduce inflammation in temporomandibular joint (TMJ) inflammation models in humans and to shorten and correct age-related delays in the resolution of acute inflammation in mice (Arnardottir et al., 2014). In the context of periodontal disease, a study in a large-animal model showed that the topical addition of a lipoxin analog, a pro-resolving nanomedicine, reduced inflammation and stimulated bone growth that was quantified by micro-computed tomography (micro-CT) (Van Dyke et al., 2015).

To find evolutionarily conserved elements of regeneration, Serhan and his team turned to planaria, a model organism that is capable of self-regeneration. Studies on the biosynthesis and actions of novel cysteinyl-specialized pro-resolving mediators in planaria head regeneration demonstrate that three pathways are activated in the resolution phase with novel mediators that are peptide–lipid conjugates (Dalli et al., 2014; de la Rosa et al., 2018). Having determined the complete stereochemistry of each of nine pathway molecules and addressed which pathways are activated in the planaria using RNA sequencing, Serhan and his team found that all three activated pathways converge on protein TRAF3 as a key player.[3] Moreover, when TRAF3 is silenced in mammalian systems, SPM actions are diminished, and the IL-10 response is lost (Chiang et al., 2021).

Together, this emerging body of evidence indicates that endogenous resolvins and SPMs activate inflammation resolution programs, said Serhan (Serhan, 2017). These mediators are intrinsic controllers of infection, are not immunosuppressant, and can help to lower antibiotic doses. Moreover, they stimulate tissue regeneration, as demonstrated in the planaria study. These data suggest the potential for these pro-resolving mediators in regenerative therapies, he added.

---

[3] TRAF3 is the tumor necrosis factor receptor-associated factor 3. It is an adaptor protein and considered a "gatekeeper" of certain immune signaling pathways (Chiang et al., 2021).

## DISCUSSION

### Characteristics of Senescent Cells

Kerr relayed a question about whether senescent stem cells could differentiate, and if so, whether the progeny would carry the senescent phenotype. Kirkland clarified that senescent cells do not divide and exist in a type of dys-differentiated state. They produce factors that impair or impede normal differentiation of cells nearby. Moreover, they can interfere with or accelerate differentiation of different types of cells that are non-senescent. In the context of bone, for example, senescent cells produce factors that can stimulate formation of osteoclasts, which resorb bone, and inhibit formation of osteoblasts, which build new bone. The combination of increasing cells that remove bone and decreasing cells that make new bone appears to contribute to age-related osteoporosis and is being explored in ongoing trials. The same effect holds in progenitors across different systems, he noted. For instance, senescent cells interfere with the differentiated state of adipose cells; fat tissue becomes insulin-resistant as a result. Senescent cells that have a pro-apoptotic SASP also interfere with differentiation of multiple other cell types. Other senescent cells, called "helper" senescent cells, can produce SASP factors (e.g., platelet-derived growth factor-AA) with beneficial effects that can improve wound healing. These types of senescent cells are not targeted by senolytics, but they are targeted in the transgenic p16 depletion mouse models.

Elisseeff added that stem cells can proliferate or they can differentiate. She posited that senescent cells could be considered simply as a differentiation state in a signaling cell. That is, the cells are signaling and communicating with the immune system to create a particular immune environment. She and her colleagues have observed this phenomenon in cartilage, and it reduces tissue production. With this perspective, a stimulus such as an infection in the body could be a signal to not make new tissue. Moreover, senescent cells may be part of the immune rheostat, which determines whether to fight a problem like infection or repair tissue, she said. Kerr added that it would be valuable to further explore the distinction between "good" and "bad" senescence and identify markers to distinguish the two. Elisseeff and her colleagues have used computational techniques to transfer the senescence signature from a transgenic animal to both mouse and human datasets, potentially revealing good-versus-bad senescence cell types and clusters. The results suggest that good types of senescence are associated with angiogenesis-like properties, whereas bad types have properties of fibrosis.

## In Vitro Systems to Investigate Senescent Cells

Kirkland was asked if in vitro systems can be used to generate and study senescent cells. He replied that senescent cells can be studied in a range of ways, including in vitro, in vivo, using tissue explants, and so forth. These cells occur across all vertebrate species, with correlates in invertebrate species as well. They are generated in response to multiple kinds of damage signals, including not only aging but also mechanical stress (e.g., in the knee joint with osteoarthritis, or shear stress) and infections of various types. For example, coronavirus can drive cells into senescence, as can bacterial, fungal, and pathogen-associated signals. Intracellular and extracellular damage can also drive senescence. Through mitochondrial communication among cells, senescence can spread through mitochondrial mechanisms as in primitive prokaryotic colonies.

## The Senescence Profile and Immunologically Induced Senescence

Kirkland was asked about the long-term effects of the senescence profile on the extracellular matrix, the associated immunological effects, and whether senolytic agents could reverse tissue-level changes. The SASP is complex, varies across different senescent cell types, and evolves over time depending upon the nature of the induced senescence, he explained. Among SASP factors are extracellular matrix proteases, MMPs, and other components that can damage the extracellular matrix. The SASP also contains large amounts of TGF-beta and activin A–related family members that result in fibrosis, as well as various types of micro RNAs that bring in different cell types that can influence the matrix. Furthermore, depending on the senescent cell type, these cells can produce a huge range of chemokines that can attract, activate, and anchor different kinds of immune cells. Senescent cells can do substantial remodeling to the extracellular matrix, he noted. The combination of senolytics and antifibrotics can, therefore, be synergistic in treating disease states associated with fibrosis such as idiopathic pulmonary fibrosis, heart failure with preserved ejection fraction, kidney disease, cirrhosis, sclerosing cholangitis, and a range of other conditions. Clinical trials will soon begin investigating these combinations for treating various kinds of conditions, he added.

Elisseeff commented that aging extracellular matrix can stiffen due not to fibrosis but to loss of proteoglycans with aging. Computational work on senescence has highlighted a role for CCN proteins that are connected to the cytoskeleton.[4] Stiffer materials in the extracellular matrix can induce senescence faster; they increase the recruitment of immune cells, such as

---

[4] For more information about CCN proteins, see Jun and Lau, 2011.

neutrophils and IL-17–producing cells, which also accelerate the onset of senescence. Macrophage cocultures with senescent cells induce more of the receptors and chemokines that communicate with T cells, demonstrating the extent of cell–cell communication between senescent cells and macrophages. The multidirectional communication is complex with T cells influencing the macrophage phenotype. Ongoing mapping efforts seek to clarify the nature and structure of these networks of communication between cell types.

Elisseeff was asked whether IL-17 induces immunosenescence globally or in specific immune cells. Immunosenescence is very different from senescence induction of certain immune phenotypes, she said. She and her colleagues are looking at senescent cell–inducing IL-17 production by various cell types. They have also observed IL-17–producing cells and IL-17–inducing cells that were fibroblasts that were previously healthy, which they refer to as an immunologically induced senescence.

## Impact of Mechanics on Response to Biomaterials

Elisseeff was asked about the role of mechanics of biomaterials to shift or otherwise affect the balance between repair and fibrosis—for example, whether immune cell infiltration could be modulated by regulating pore sizes in implanted materials. Indeed, shape, porosity, and mechanics of the materials can influence the response, she said. For instance, stiffer hydrogels are associated with more fibrosis, greater numbers of neutrophils, and different macrophage phenotypes. These mechanical properties can be modulated, as evidenced in recent papers about the impact of the surface topography of breast implants on fibrosis and serious adverse events in patients. The systemic state of the patient is also relevant and can change over time, Elisseeff added. For example, a patient might receive a cosmetic filler without initial reaction and then have a sudden fibrotic inflammatory response months after injection, which may be due to a systemic change that modulates the local response. Considerations about how the systemic state of an individual may influence the response to injury—with or without a biomaterial—are important from clinical and patient-centered perspectives, she suggested.

## Timing of Immune Response Resolution

Serhan was asked about the window of opportunity to capture the resolution of the immune response, processes that took 12–24 hours in the studies he presented. Specifically, he was asked if a short timeframe is common or universal across different tissues or methods of stem cell transplants. Serhan replied that the timing operates differently at each site of inflammation and in an organ-dependent manner. In the work he presented, the ideal timing was modeled with respect to an inflammatory exudate. With other published animal models, even treatment at the maximum time of the inflammatory response could help trigger endogenous resolution. Thus, the timing and dose of the intervention must be tailored to each system independently, he said. Resolvins, lipoxin analogs, and mimetics have been shown to increase survival in animal models of transplants, Serhan added, which is encouraging and may offer opportunities to synergize with some of the mechanisms discussed by the other presenters.

### Applications and Mechanisms of Pro-resolving Mediators

Kerr asked about the mechanisms that the resolvins target within stem cells themselves, and whether they target quiescent cells or replicative stem cells. Serhan and his colleagues have shown that stem cells produce pro-resolving mediators, as well as prostaglandins and other factors. While other research groups have demonstrated the signal transduction, his group elucidated the receptor themselves. The receptors are present on various stem cells, but after the receptor–ligand interaction, the cellular mechanisms of action are highly cell-type-dependent.

Kerr inquired about the effects of immune response manipulation on stem progenitor cells. Serhan and his lab have demonstrated that periodontal stem cells produce pro-resolving mediators and that these mediators act on neural stem cells. Advances made by other research groups are also promising, including the recent publication demonstrating that resolvin D2 stimulates muscle regeneration, which has the potential for treating Duchenne muscular dystrophy (Dort et al., 2021).

Serhan was also asked what happens if neutrophils or macrophages are absent or blocked, and whether it would be effective to add mediators of their function. He replied that it is unlikely that the complex role of the macrophage—particularly the M2 macrophage—or the neutrophil could be substituted by a single mediator that they produce or that acts on them. However, if they are absent from the system, other targets have been elucidated for pro-resolving mediators, and their receptors appear in other tissues, representing opportunities for future study.

### Manipulation of Immune Responses and Autoimmunity Issues

Kerr asked about any concerns or evidence that manipulating immune responses might generate autoimmunity issues. Elisseeff replied that the corollary of that question is whether manipulating immune responses can be used to treat autoimmune disease in new ways. The IL-17 signature, for instance, is associated with certain autoimmune diseases such as psoriatic arthritis. Resolving a wound in various ways could also help determine the signatures of autoimmunity. There are potential benefits of manipulating immune responses as well as dangers, she said. Serhan added that evidence is emerging about the effects of resolvins on autoimmunity for osteoarthritis and rheumatoid arthritis, for example, in which the administration of resolvins appears to result in a diminished inflammatory response and improved cartilage production and function. He suggested that there are many opportunities to consider the appropriate indications and disease scenarios to deliver pro-resolving mediators, which is why his group has used planaria to investigate highly conserved components of tissue regeneration that intersect with the actions of pro-resolving mediators.

# 7

# Tools and Preclinical Models for Monitoring and Optimizing the Host's Pro-Regenerative Environment

---

**Key Points Highlighted by Individual Speakers**

- Cellular neighborhoods are defined as repeatable units of different cell types found in tissues and the immune system. Some structures are tissue specific, and others are conserved across different tissues. (Nolan)
- Interfaces between cellular neighborhoods reveal information about the local biology and may have prognostic value. (Nolan)
- CD19-targeted chimeric antigen receptor (CAR) immunotherapies use engineered T cells with synthetic receptors to treat certain types of cancer; these cells can be designed and manufactured as "living drugs." (Sadelain)
- Novel applications of CAR T-cell therapies for regenerative medicine may include removing senescent cells and modulating tissue regeneration. (Sadelain)
- To create targeted therapeutics and develop rationally designed biomaterials, it is important to consider and interrogate the underlying basic biology. Multidisciplinary studies that integrate this knowledge across fields will push the field of regenerative medicine forward. (Sadtler)
- Future research should make use of integrative, iterative approaches that apply preclinical and quantitative modeling results to clinical data and vice versa. (Sadtler)

The fifth session of the workshop explored the development of tools and preclinical models for monitoring and optimizing the host's pro-regenerative environment. The objectives of this session were to (1) explore recent advances in monitoring and imaging of the immune system as well as the potential implications of these new approaches for clinical translation of regenerative medicines and (2) discuss challenges and opportunities with regard to preclinical models for studying immune system involvement in response to regenerative medicine. The session was moderated by Sadik Kassim of Vor Biopharma.

## TOOLS FOR IMMUNE PROFILING AND MONITORING

Garry Nolan, Rachford and Carlota Harris Professor in the Department of Pathology at Stanford University, discussed how new multiplex tools can be used for immune profiling and monitoring, with a particular focus on cancer. Tissue damage initiates wound repair, a type of disruption that provides insight into the rules that underpin tissue architecture, he commented. The immune system is intimately involved in wound repair, which is a highly dynamic process involving cellular rearrangement. Thus, a view of the immune system as a dynamic and mobile organ is an instructive starting point, he said. Multiple tools are now available, such as mass cytometry and imaging versions of single-cell analysis: multiplexing, ion beam imaging, and a new split-pool approach with potential to substantially reduce the cost of single-cell RNA and protein analysis and ATAC-Seq,[1] Nolan described. At the most fundamental level, this work is about the tissue architecture as defined not only by the cell–cell interactions but also by the tissue context. Until recently, the tools and mathematics to understand those issues have not been available. "Tissue building blocks"—also called "tissue schematics"—can be used to elucidate the essential rules of the immune system's operation in both normal and pathologic circumstances, which can then be used to extract meaning and (eventually) identify therapeutic targets, Nolan explained.

### CODEX: CO-Detection by indEXing Tool for Multiplex Imaging by Reannealing

Nolan and his team developed the CO-Detection by indEXing (CODEX) multiplexing microscopy tool, which is based on reannealing groups of oligo-fluorophores to precisely image tissues and characterize cell types (Goltsev et al., 2018). The CODEX approach is relatively straightforward and consists of several steps, Nolan explained. The first step is to stain

---

[1] Assay for Transposase-Accessible Chromatin with high-throughput sequencing.

with 50–120 antibodies, each of which has a unique DNA tag. In groups of three, oligonucleotides, each of which is antisense to a DNA-labeled individual antibody and has a unique fluorophore label, are annealed, and then imaging is conducted at the desired level of resolution. Next, the oligonucleotides are removed by simple denaturation, and subsequent sets of oligo-fluorophores are annealed and imaged iteratively. The process is performed by a robot that moves the reagents and the oligonucleotides into different chambers where the chemistry occurs. Advantages of the CODEX approach include its integration with existing microscope platforms, making it broadly accessible to more researchers, and that it does not require coordinating with a tissue analysis core, he said.

In the current era, collecting data through the CODEX approach and analysis methods is relatively straightforward; rather, the primary challenges are data analysis and extraction of meaning from large datasets, Nolan remarked. In the context of cancer, the CODEX tool is more predictive due to the insight acquired into how cells are organized, which is more instructive than any individual set of markers identified using simpler modalities (Lu et al., 2019). For instance, adding multiplex immunohistochemistry to other datasets—such as gene expression profiling, programmed death-ligand 1 (PD-L1) immunohistochemistry, and tumor mutation burden—can yield a higher area under the curve (AUC) in ROC curve analysis (Lu et al., 2019).[2] It may also be especially informative to combine a multiplexing microscopy tool like CODEX with traditional RNA sequencing analysis.

To date, the CODEX system has more than 130 validated DNA-barcoded human antibodies (Bhate et al., 2021; Hickey et al., 2021; Phillips et al., 2021; Schurch et al., 2020). Nolan explained that they start by identifying high-level phenotyping markers that distinguish well-known cell types, as well as tissue-specific or intracellular markers, such as phospho-specific markers. These markers are used to further define both the cell phenotype and the activation state (e.g., if the cell is dividing, whether it has recently seen an antigen) based on whether those markers are positive or not in a given cell.

## Cellular Neighborhoods

Nolan introduced the model framework of cellular neighborhoods (CNs) to explain how the CODEX tool can be used to understand cancer and other pathologies. CNs are defined by a characteristic local composition of cell types. In neighborhood analysis, an analysis window passes across CODEX-derived images of tissue to assess the composition of cell

---

[2] Receiver operating characteristic (ROC) curve analysis is a classical method of evaluating the predictive success of a classification model.

types present based on standardized cell determinations and established algorithms. If a set of cell types is found repeatedly across a unit, it is defined as a neighborhood, and tissues typically have 10–15 CNs (Bhate et al., 2021; Phillips et al., 2021; Schurch et al., 2020). These CNs typically coincide nicely with what pathologists are accustomed to seeing with traditional histology, Nolan noted. The next steps of analysis are to (1) examine how the different CNs interact with each other; (2) identify any rules by which they interact, not only as neighborhoods but as cells within the neighborhood; and (3) explore whether there is anything distinct about the interface between CNs.

A variety of mathematical approaches can be applied to determine whether there are standardized rules and interactions that seem to be obvious between cells (Schurch et al., 2020). The interactions themselves are not observed as such; rather, they are inferred based on repeated behavior or the repeated incidence of cell context, which implies the potential importance of the cell's presence (or not), Nolan elaborated. When the data indicate an interaction exists, Nolan and his colleagues search for literature evidence to support the proposed interaction and apply advanced statistical methods (e.g., tensor analysis) to derive meaning from it. One of the objectives of this process is to determine whether there are CNs, or cell types within neighborhoods, that might predict survival outcomes or some other mechanistic determination, said Nolan. Importantly, this work extends beyond mapping to extract information about underlying dynamic behavior from a static image, he emphasized. The various types of inter-CN relationships give rise to the most compelling aspect of this research because the relationships may broaden understanding of how changes in the dynamic processes that underlie pathology relate to a positive or negative resolution, Nolan remarked.

### Lymph Node Cellular Neighborhoods

To demonstrate how relational rules can be extracted from CN analysis, Nolan used the example of lymph nodes from the tonsil and spleen, because they provide a standard baseline of a nonactivated immune system. The lymph nodes across the human body are evolutionarily similar, yet the tissues have structural differences, he noted. Conducting a CN analysis on those lymph nodes revealed about ten different neighborhoods, identified based on the primary cell type (e.g., granulocytes, B cells, T cells, macrophages) that seems to be reflective of the neighborhood itself (Schurch et al., 2020). Although the overall set of CNs is similar across lymph node subtypes, within a particular CN, differences in the presence or absence of various cell types can be identified, thereby providing means to distinguish between the lymph node subtypes (Schurch et al., 2020).

To determine rules from cellular relationships, the next step is to consider each CN and identify how it relates to other neighborhoods by identifying common and unique adjacencies. These rules can be used to build a tree structure to visualize observable inter-CN relationships that seem to be repeated within individual lymph node types (Schurch et al., 2020). Some rules are common across the various lymph nodes. There are tissue-specific structures as well as evolutionarily conserved structures that seem to be present or necessary across all the different lymph node types, Nolan emphasized. These rules are then used to examine whether those same types of structures also occur surreptitiously or adventitiously in pathology tissue in the case of cancer, for example.

*Case Study: Colorectal Tumor Immune Microenvironment*

To illustrate how cellular neighborhoods can be used to study pathology, Nolan and his team conducted a case study of the colorectal tumor immune microenvironment (Schurch et al., 2020). For the study, they narrowed down a large cohort of colorectal patients to identify two extreme classes of disease that are associated with different patient outcomes, Nolan explained. One category included patients with a diffuse inflammatory infiltrate that appears disorganized and who tend to have poor outcomes. The second category was characterized by Crohn's-like reactions, in which a follicle is visible, with an immune system infiltrate that seems organized; this group of patients is associated with better outcomes.

For each tumor, a pathologist examined the tumor–immune interface to distinguish different ecosystems that might represent the total ecosystem of the tumor, stated Nolan. Four samples from each tumor were analyzed in a tumor microarray to search for rules. Researchers stained with approximately 60 markers, determined the cell types, and conducted neighborhood analysis. The initial expectation was that the two classes of tumors would have very different neighborhoods; surprisingly, this did not prove to be the case, he said. Regardless of how the tumors were clustered, the same kinds of neighborhoods were observed; however, the organization of the neighborhoods was extremely different, he explained. In patients that do poorly, CNs exhibit fragmentation, suggesting that the immune system is not allowed to become organized. This insight may be valuable in the context of tissue regeneration, he added. For example, there may be instances of pathology in which the immune system is unable to form a coherent structure that would enable it to carry out its function.

Nolan and his colleagues initially focused on whether they could relate any kind of cell-type observations to cancer outcome. In short, the presence or absence of certain cell types in the tissue was not reflective of outcome. However, investigating the presence or absence of certain cell types within certain definable neighborhoods suddenly revealed an entire litany of relationships that were positively or negatively predictive of patient outcome. Thus, cell type matters, but cell type in a particular context matters more, Nolan emphasized.

The final step in this process is to organize the observations into relationships to determine how the cell types are organized relative to each other. Specifically, the interfaces between neighborhoods and the changes in the cell types of those neighborhoods reflect the biology, so the upregulation of cells at the interface is just as important as the presence or absence of the cell type, explained Nolan. The CN interfaces provide information about the biology that enables a specialist with domain knowledge to determine what they mean locally. Furthermore, this organizational information has prognostic value and can become reflective of a prediction and an outcome, Nolan said. Local CNs and the relationships between them can be used to predict which type of tumor a patient has, which may influence therapeutic options, he suggested. In the context of regenerative medicine, mapping the organization of pathologies could inform the development of novel therapeutics to enhance tissue regeneration processes.

## ENGINEERED IMMUNITY AS A MODEL FOR REGENERATIVE MEDICINE

Michel Sadelain, Stephen and Barbara Friedman Chair and Director of the Center for Cell Engineering at the Memorial Sloan Kettering Cancer Center, discussed therapeutic tools with potential applications in the field of regenerative medicine.

### Mastering T-Cell Responses

Novel immunotherapeutic tools emerged with the rise of engineered T cells as cancer drugs. T cells engineered with a chimeric antigen receptor can delay tumor progression and, importantly, be a curative modality, Sadelain remarked. Realizing this curative potential requires mastering several fundamental components of biology: (1) how to harness T-cell specificity, (2) how to support the functional persistence of T cells, and (3) how to achieve the potency needed to overcome tumors and the tumor microenvironment.

T cells form in the thymus, where they acquire their T-cell receptors (Janeway et al., 2001). The T-cell receptor is generated through the recombination of hundreds of genes that can form a vast number of potential T-cell receptors, Sadelain explained. The repertoire of receptors is pruned as it is formed to obey the laws of immune tolerance, with the average adult human harboring an estimated 20 million different specificities (Chen et al., 2017).

The medical field has long attempted to direct the T-cell repertoire through a range of approaches. The most well-established strategy is active immunization, which involves trying to amplify a subset of T cells that would protect against a future infectious disease. A more recent approach, harnessed specifically in the domain of cancer, is known as checkpoint blockade immunotherapy, which uses antibodies to relieve inhibition on tumor-reactive T cells. A third approach, chimeric antigen receptor (CAR) T-cell engineering, employs genetic engineering to instruct T-cell functionality and is the primary focus of Sadelain's work.

### Assembling Chimeric Antigen Receptors for Cell Therapy

Sadelain provided an overview of the process by which CARs, or synthetic T-cell receptors, are assembled for cell therapy (Riviere and Sadelain, 2017). Incorporating knowledge from tumor biology and the immunology of T cells, the approach is heavily predicated on genetic engineering and takes advantage of an expanding array of tools to modify T cells with synthetic receptors. CARs substitute for physiologic antigen receptors (i.e., T-cell receptors) to instruct the function of engineered T cells, he explained. Rather than engage human leukocyte antigen (HLA) peptide complexes as the normal adaptive immune system does, CARs engage cell surface molecules like CD19.[3] Given initial skepticism about the potential value of this form of immunotherapy, academic investigators had to develop their own cell-manufacturing sciences to introduce genes into T cells and regulate them up to FDA standards, Sadelain said. At the outset of the manufacturing process, T cells were typically retrieved from a patient through apheresis. The cells were then genetically modified as they were activated and slightly expanded, quality controlled, released, and infused back to the recipient (Hollyman et al., 2009).

### Clinical History and Impact of CD19 CAR Therapy

The CD19 paradigm demonstrated the therapeutic potential of CAR immunotherapy in the clinic, Sadelain observed. The two first CARs for immunotherapy were approved by the FDA in 2017 to treat certain B-cell malignancies: CD28 CAR (axicabtagene ciloleucel) and 4-1BB CAR (tisagenlecleucel). Both prototypical CARs are specific for the molecule CD19, which had been previously identified as a potential target for CARs (Brentjens et al., 2003). Both CARs comprise an array of signaling domains that are not normally found on the same molecule. The molecular structures

---

[3] CD19 is a transmembrane protein expressed by normal B cells until differentiation and by most B-cell malignancies (Hollyman et al., 2009).

include an activation domain and one or more costimulatory domains that further amplify the signal and impart a different functional profile to the genetically enhanced cells (Maher et al., 2002), Sadelain elaborated. Three clinical trials that were conducted at three separate academic medical centers established the therapeutic value of the first CD19 CARs by demonstrating rapid and complete eradication of refractory leukemia by 1928z CAR T cells (Brentjens et al., 2013; Couzin-Frankel, 2013; June and Sadelain, 2018). Sadelain highlighted several major clinical impacts of CD19 CAR therapy, the first gene therapy to be approved in the United States and the first engineered T cell to be approved worldwide (see Box 7-1). Perhaps most importantly, the success of the CD19 treatment paradigm convinced the pharmaceutical and biotechnology sectors to contemplate manufacturing cells as drugs, moving beyond chemicals to pave the path forward for novel cellular therapeutics, he said.

Today, work on developing these types of therapies has expanded to the extent that 700 CAR trials are listed at ClinicalTrials.Gov as of March 2021, with 40 percent of those targeting CD19 (Globerson Levin et al., 2021). This percentage is likely to decrease over time as new targets are brought to bear, Sadelain predicted. Yet, many researchers still choose to include CD19 in initial tests of new manufacturing strategies, CAR designs, molecules, or combinations of molecules. He added that the vast majority (about 95 percent) of interventional CAR clinical trials are being conducted in the United States and China (MacKay et al., 2020).

## Therapeutic Potential of Senolytic CAR T Cells in Regenerative Medicine

In addition to providing a paradigm for the development of CAR T cells, advances in CD19 CAR therapy have potential to open new avenues

---

**BOX 7-1**
**Impacts of CD19 CAR Therapy**

- Provides clinical benefit for patients with relapsed B-cell malignancies
- Ushered "synthetic biology" (e.g., chimeric proteins) into the clinical arena
- Convinced Big Pharma to manufacture cells as medicines (i.e., "living drugs")
- Catalyzed rethinking drug manufacturing, distribution, and reimbursement
- Poised to extend to other cancers and pathologies
- Paves the way for other cell and gene therapies

SOURCE: Sadelain presentation, November 3, 2021.

for other cell therapies, said Sadelain. These include therapies targeting other hematological malignancies (e.g., myeloma, acute myeloid leukemia), solid tumors, severe infections, and autoimmunity or even inducing tolerance in organ transplantation.

CAR T cells also have prospective applications in regenerative medicine, Sadelain said. Specifically, while investigating the potential to use CAR T cells to remove senescent cells, he and his team conducted a search for surface molecules induced by senescence and identified the urokinase plasminogen activator receptor (uPAR) as a means to target senescent cells (Amor et al., 2020). Since CARs engage molecules (e.g., proteins, carbohydrates, glycolipids) on the cell surface, the researchers examined the surface profiles of cells induced into senescence through a variety of stress triggers and found that the protein uPAR is a biomarker of senescence. In various murine models that induce senescence and fibrosis in the liver, a single infusion of senolytic CAR T cells targeted to uPAR not only removed the senescent cells but also restored tissue homeostasis in senescence-associated fibrosis (Amor et al., 2020; Wagner and Gil, 2020).

Senolytic CAR T cells thus represent a novel tool to leverage the engineering of immune cells—including T cells but also natural killer cells, macrophages, or perhaps neutrophils—by targeting them through genetic engineering, assessing their function on clearance of senescent cells, and evaluating their ability to facilitate or induce organ regeneration, Sadelain suggested. Regenerative medicine can reciprocally offer new prospects for the development of tools and therapies to the field of T-cell engineering, he noted. For instance, CAR therapy typically relies on autologous T cells collected from patients, but investigators are interested in alternatives like collecting cells from healthy volunteers or using pluripotent stem cells. The field of regenerative medicine has generated knowledge about working with these cell types that could also serve the development of CAR therapies.

*Generation of CAR T Cell In Vitro from Pluripotent Stem Cells*

In 2013, Sadelain and his group provided a first proof of concept that the CAR T cells could be generated in vitro starting from pluripotent stem cells (Themeli et al., 2013). They were able to reprogram T cells to a pluripotent state or ground-state level, introduce therein a CAR that was constitutively expressed, and then re-induce lymphoid populations from these pluripotent stem cells. They have since made considerable progress in defining the requirements for these differentiations, he noted.

The induction of T cells from pluripotent stem cells is not straightforward because T cells are not uniform and acquire different properties that define distinct lineages or commitments in their fate, explained Sadelain. Furthermore, this differentiation is dictated by the T-cell receptor that is uniquely acquired in every clonotype. Despite these complexities, methods like single-cell RNA studies can now elucidate the sequence of steps that the pluripotent stem cell undergoes until it becomes a CD8 T lymphocyte. Today, T cells can be induced to both express a CAR and no longer harbor their endogenous T-cell receptor; these cells look more like physiological CD8 T cells than gamma-delta T cells or other immune cells, Sadelain described. To further direct the fates of T cells and their corresponding therapeutic profiles, the researchers have successfully induced CD19-specific CAR T cells that display a phenotype similar to effector memory T cells. These cells have exhibited therapeutic effectiveness in models of leukemia.

In the context of advancing regenerative medicine, Sadelain emphasized a key lesson from the development of CD19 CAR therapy. The field of cell therapy is no longer limited to isolating and expanding naturally occurring T cells. Instead, it is feasible to begin considering design and manufacturing approaches for (1) overcoming immune tolerance, (2) dictating to T cells which antigens to recognize, and (3) controlling their effector functions and durability in vivo. In closing, Sadelain expressed his hope that these tools will be of use to advance regenerative medicine.

## BASIC IMMUNOLOGY TO GUIDE REGENERATIVE THERAPEUTIC DESIGN

Kaitlyn Sadtler, Earl Stadtman Tenure-Track Investigator and chief of the Section on Immunoengineering at the National Institute of Biomedical Imaging and Bioengineering, discussed how basic immunology can guide regenerative therapeutic design, noting that it is now possible to apply an understanding of mechanistic biology to guide the design of biomaterials.

### Immunoengineering in Human Health and Disease

The various functions of the immune system in human health and disease give rise to the potential of immunoengineering (i.e., engineering the immune system) to promote health, Sadtler remarked. In addition to playing a critical role in defense against pathogens, the immune system recognizes and responds to implanted materials from medical devices (e.g., breast implant, hip replacement) through the foreign body response, she explained. In the context of wound healing, the immune system determines whether scar tissue is formed or functional tissue is regenerated. Therefore, engineering the immune system can have broad impact across a variety of fields including tissue engineering and regenerative medicine, but also cancer therapeutics, autoimmunity, medical device design, and others, she said.

### Scaffold Immune Microenvironment

The tumor immunology field developed the concept of an immune microenvironment, which has now been adopted by other fields, Sadtler remarked. The immune microenvironment of a biomaterial scaffold can alter the proliferation and differentiation of stem and progenitor cells. Her laboratory and others are looking more deeply into the immune response to the injury and to the material implantation. Both the location of an injury and the type of implanted material can affect immune cell recruitment, activation, and polarization, creating a varied repertoire of different cells and signaling molecules that can then ultimately interact with stem cells, explained Sadtler. In a pro-regenerative environment, this can lead to functional tissue development. Alternatively, an adverse environment could cause pathologic outcomes, such as excessive inflammation or fibrotic scarring.

### Immune Cell Polarization

Polarization of immune cells is the process by which components of the immune system (e.g., macrophages, T cells) functionalize to home in on the right response to the challenge at hand, Sadtler explained. Importantly, the appropriate response in one situation may not be appropriate in another situation. For example, "good" type 1 inflammation can clear virally infected cells to prevent the spread of infection whereas "bad" type 1 inflammation can prevent proper healing, she elaborated. Similarly, "good" type 2 inflammation can promote extracellular matrix deposition and muscle wound healing, but "bad" type 2 inflammation can result in pathogenic scarring and thick fibrotic scar tissue deposition.

### Biologically Oriented Therapeutic Development

Developing specific, targeted therapeutics depends upon an understanding of basic biology and relying on biology as the foundation from which to create rationally designed materials from the bottom up, Sadtler suggested. A prime example of engineering the immune system based on understanding biology is checkpoint blockade immunotherapy, she noted. By understanding the basic biology of how T cells regulate their responses to prevent overreaction, engineers and biologists created a therapeutic that could block these interactions in patients with tumors that pathologically upregulated the suppressive responses. In the context of wound healing, understanding the biology of how the body responds to biomaterial implants could be used to develop targeted therapeutics. Sadtler emphasized that such work requires multidisciplinary effort that integrates knowledge across fields (e.g., wound healing, developmental biology, stem cell biology, immunology, materials science, bioengineering, chemistry).

## Modeling the Poles of Innate Immune Responses with Representative Materials

To evaluate immune responses to implanted biomaterials, Sadtler and her team model opposing "poles" of immune responses using two representative materials—one pro-fibrotic and one pro-regenerative—implanted in a mouse model. The pro-fibrotic material is polyethylene, which is highly hydrophobic and nondegradable, and produces constant inflammation and fibrosis. The pro-regenerative material is extracellular matrix (ECM), which is biologically derived and degradable, and used clinically in hernia repair, dural repair, and diabetic ulcers. ECM scaffolds have even shown promise in complex trauma repair like muscle injury, she noted. In comparing the two poles of immune responses, there is a clear shift among granulocytes from a neutrophil-dominant phenotype in a pro-fibrotic or pro-inflammatory material to an eosinophil-dominant response in the ECM material (Sadtler et al., 2019). Eosinophils (Siglec-F+ cells) are present in type 2 immune responses, such as allergies, and neutrophils (Ly6G+ cells) are characteristic of viral and bacterial infections, she added.

Other laboratories have also advanced the understanding of these phenotypes, said Sadtler. Ed Botchwey and his team, for example, have identified functionally diverse subpopulations of neutrophils that respond to tissue defects (Turner et al., 2020). In a project led by Josh Doloff, Bob Langer's research group showed that macrophages—but not neutrophils—were required for fibrosis in the foreign body response and that a macrophage inhibitor could reduce fibrosis (Doloff et al., 2017). Finally, James Anderson and his colleagues published seminal work on the role of macrophages in fibrotic foreign body responses to biomaterials (Anderson et al., 2008).

## Role of T Cells in Adaptive Immunity

Expanding their considerations from innate to adaptive immunity, Sadtler and her colleagues also examined the role of T cells in wound healing and found that interleukin 4 (IL-4) upregulation is dependent upon adaptive immune cells, especially CD4+ cells (Sadtler et al., 2016).[4] In the context of muscle injury and pro-regenerative biomaterials, the loss of adaptive immune cells—specifically Th2 cells and the protein IL-4—leads to (1) a loss of a pro-regenerative macrophage phenotype and (2) a massive

---

[4] CD4+ cells are a subtype of helper T cells (Sadtler et al., 2016).

imbalance in cell differentiation and muscle healing (Sadtler et al., 2016). In mouse models without adaptive immune cells, small, irregularly shaped muscle fibers and substantial intramuscular adipose deposits are observed after a muscle injury, described Sadtler. The phenotype can be rescued by supplementing mice that lack an adaptive immune system with wild-type T cells. However, if the supplemental T cells cannot polarize via the Th2 pathway, the pro-regenerative phenotype is not rescued; establishing Th2-specific polarization is required, she emphasized.

Sadtler highlighted other efforts to explore the role of adaptive immunity in wound healing. For instance, Ajay Chawla's research group found that eosinophil activation and type 2 immune signals were necessary for muscle regeneration after a cardiotoxin injury (Heredia et al., 2013). Steve Badylak and his colleagues demonstrated that ECM integration into a muscle defect correlated with the presence of M2 polarized macrophages (Badylak et al., 2008). Bryan Brown's lab modified polymers to elute IL-4 to promote implant integration and minimize type 1 inflammation at the site of implant (Hachim et al., 2017). Dave Mooney and his team showed that IL-4–functionalized gold nanoparticles could promote the recovery of muscle after injury (Raimondo and Mooney, 2018).

### Human Immune Responses to Trauma and Recovery: Learning from Clinical Data

While the context of mouse models can be useful, Sadtler emphasized the importance of learning from clinical models and patients to inform animal models of disease, and vice versa. For a large biomarkers study, her team is building a database of clinical data to evaluate the systemic immune status of patients at admission for various types of traumas. Researchers can use the database to consider demographic information that correlates with trauma outcome, identify proteins that might predict recovery, and inform the design of biomaterials for treatment of an injury. Other laboratories have also explored biomarkers and large datasets to better understand the injury environment, she added. Garry Nolan and his team used a computational approach to identify different cell types associated with surgical recovery (Gaudilliere et al., 2014). Robert Guldberg and his colleagues detected biomarkers that correlated with bone regeneration after trauma (Cheng et al., 2021), while Jennifer Elisseeff's research group utilized single-cell sequencing to define new immune cell subpopulations in response to biomaterials (Sommerfeld et al., 2019).

## Examining the Future of Immunoengineering and Regenerative Therapeutic Design

Sadtler underscored the importance of applying basic biology and integrating various types of data to guide regenerative therapeutic design. To create better therapeutics, it may be valuable to consider the existing approach to solving these fundamental problems, how studies are currently designed, and how to untangle the basic biology to learn from the immune system, she explained. Given animal models and a set of preliminary materials, it is possible to assess the tissue structure and the basic immunology of the materials as well as apply computational approaches to further study them. This information can be aggregated in a database of known responses and outcomes and applied to the clinical development of materials; that clinical knowledge can also augment development of preclinical models, she said. Eventually, the aim would be to start with quantitative modeling and perturb the computational system to eliminate approaches that are unlikely to be successful before testing them in vivo or in the clinic, Sadtler described.

There are multiple approaches underway to integrate these data and engineer biomaterials for immune-guided regenerative therapeutics—for example, to prevent fibrosis of the medical devices used in reconstruction and to grow back new tissues using regenerative therapeutics, she explained. Another promising avenue is to combine quantitative modeling with patient data to develop individualized therapeutics, Sadtler said. It may be possible to predict the outcome of an intervention based on the patient's biology and use in vitro platforms to evaluate therapeutic design and dosing on an individual-by-individual basis. In addition to precision medicine, which can be cost prohibitive, broad-reaching therapeutics are important for promoting human health, noted Sadtler. To drive efforts of bioengineering for human health, the National Institute of Biomedical Imaging and Bioengineering recently announced the launch of the Center for Biomedical Engineering and Technology Acceleration within its intramural research program. The initiative aims to drive innovative science through diverse people with diverse minds to catalyze the development of new technologies for human health.

## DISCUSSION

### Effect of Biomaterial on Immune Response

Kassim asked Sadtler to elaborate on the model she presented framing biomaterials as pro-regenerative versus pro-fibrotic. He asked if pro-regenerative biomaterial is always pro-regenerative, or whether it is context specific. Sadtler replied that it is context specific, and there are also limitations based on material properties, such as mechanics. In unpublished studies, her group compared a subcutaneous injury, a muscle injury, and an intraperitoneal implantation. The intraperitoneal implant exhibited more B-cell recruitment than the other injuries did, indicating different immune responses to the same material, she explained. Furthermore, clinical experience shows that immune response differs based on the location where a material is placed (e.g., adjacent to fat versus muscle), and some organs can sustain a more robust immune response than others, she added.

Sadtler was asked whether immune responses change when progenitor stem cells are added to biomaterials before implantation in the host. She replied that her group has not investigated that directly because their work focuses primarily on endogenous repair, but she noted that stem cells themselves can be highly immunomodulatory. For instance, MSCs are known to alter the immune response associated with a material. Sadtler added that researchers at the University of Florida have studied allogeneic encapsulated islet cells to treat type 1 diabetes and found that encapsulation of the cells altered the immune response as well (Stabler et al., 2020). Cell-laden therapeutics should be evaluated to understand how the cells and their secretome might affect surrounding immune cells, Sadtler said.

### CAR T Therapy: Conditioning and Mechanistic Functioning

Noting that lymphoid depletion and conditioning are important aspects of CAR therapy efficacy, Kassim asked Sadelain whether similar conditioning to create a receptive environment would be required for senolytic CAR treatment. Sadelain replied that conditioning—sometimes called lymphodepletion—is a key component. It is well established that T cells cannot simply be infused into an immunocompetent recipient to achieve tumor rejection; it requires some form of prior conditioning, such as a short pulse of chemotherapy. Reducing the number of host lymphocytes increases the chance that available cytokines will support the CAR T cell rather than host T cells, he said. Conditioning has many other effects, including on the endothelium and the gut, and may reduce tumor burden in some cases. Further study in humans and experimental models would be beneficial to understand optimal conditioning, Sadelain suggested.

Kassim then asked what is known about the mechanism of action of senolytic CARs. Sadelain responded that this question cannot be fully addressed yet within the nascent field of senescence, partially due to the heterogeneity of senescent cells. In terms of CAR T cells, re-engineering provides them with new means to engage a different range of targets. Accordingly, the engineered cells may not engage with antigen-presenting cells because they do not recognize HLA; rather, their action is more restricted to the intended target. He added that with genetic engineering and other tools "we're starting to bend the rules" to develop novel therapeutics.

### Role of Costimulatory Domains in Modulating the Function of CAR T Cells

Sadelain was asked about differences in costimulatory domains to modulate the function of CAR T cells for immune suppression, specifically with respect to regulatory T cells compared to antitumor CAR T cells or senolytic CAR T cells. He explained that the costimulatory domain is critical in shaping and programming functions into an engineered T cell, the most classical being the two canonical CARs that use either the CD28 or the 41BB costimulatory domain. The CD28 domain creates an "explosive" effector cell endowed with maximal effector functions, but this comes at the expense of longevity of the cells, which rapidly proceed into terminal differentiation. Other costimulatory domains, 41BB being the prototype, program a weaker effector profile, but they enhance the persistence of those cells. Research is underway to find additional costimulatory molecules that may further fine-tune the properties of therapeutic T cells, he noted.

### Comparative Morphology with Multiplexing Tools

Kassim commented that the CODEX platform has been used to perform comparative morphology between mouse and man. He asked about any themes that have emerged from this work, such as similarities between the neighborhoods of mouse and human spleens—and about the extent to which mouse models can be used to derive fundamental observations about the human CNs. Nolan replied that his group has comparatively analyzed models from human and primate to mouse. Although there were individualized differences, at a global level, the CNs were relatively similar, so based on this work, they are beginning to use neighborhoods to define the functional correspondence of cell types across species, he said. He noted that these results follow the same premise as the tissue disorganization observed in certain kinds of cancers. Together, these studies suggest a fundamental rule of tissue organization; his group is working to determine other basic rules and how they may be altered to serve a pathologic function.

### Composition of Cellular Neighborhoods within the Same Tumor Type

Nolan was asked whether he and his lab have observed any differences in the composition of CNs of the same tumor type in an individual patient. He said that they have not investigated this in patients but considered a related question in a mouse model of melanoma. If a lymph node is analyzed before a tumor enters the tissue, there are no differences in the cell types. However, rearrangement of the cells is detectable, which indicates either (1) the tumor signals to the lymph node ahead of its arrival or (2) the immune system already recognizes the tumor. When the tumor enters the lymph node, the cellular organization again rearranges, an effect which Nolan likened to "scattering the barstools in the saloon."

### Cellular Architecture of Immune-Desert Tumor Types

Kassim inquired about features within immune-desert tumor types that may point to unique neighborhood architectures that correlate with absence of immune infiltration. Nolan responded that they have made such observations, which appear to be driven by the presence of the tumor itself, as if the tumor creates an immune exclusion zone. It appears that when a tumor inserts itself into the tissue, it deactivates positive aspects of the immune response organization such that it creates that immune-desert environment, he said.

### Use of CODEX to Image 3D Tissues

Nolan was asked if the CODEX platform can be adapted to stain and image optically cleared three-dimensional tissues. He confirmed that it can, if the tissues are not too thick and the appropriate microscope is used. The primary challenge is that thicker tissues require more time to flush one set of oligo-fluorophores out and reanneal another set so the speed is more difficult to achieve. While some research applications may benefit from three-dimensional analysis, Nolan emphasized that the multiplexing microscopy tool in combination with the appropriate analysis methods can capture the biological dynamics of three dimensions with a simple two-dimensional slice. The next steps will be to move to a sample thickness of 50–100 microns, which would not require complex optics to process, he said.

### Developing New Tools and Preclinical Models

Kassim asked each presenter for their perspectives on priorities in developing tools and preclinical models for both monitoring the performance of regenerative medicines and using them to create more effective therapies. In the context of early-stage translational science, Sadtler discussed the potential benefits of collecting more clinical data and conducting more thorough analyses of human responses to materials and trauma. The integration of knowledge across various fields working on relevant biology will be important moving forward, she predicted. For example, different fields have worked on immunology in various contexts such as scarring and skin wound healing or type 2 immune responses to multicellular parasites. A lot can be gained from bringing together investigators from different specialties, she said.

Sadelain encouraged the development of a cell-based approach to treat conditions that are secondary to the accumulation or poor removal of senescent cells. In both the expanding field of senolytics and other disciplines, there is a tendency to focus on developing highly specific molecular interventions, and chemicals as drugs are enticing due to their convenience, he observed. However, a cell-based approach may be more suitable in the context of complex phenomena, including those explored during the workshop. In those types of phenomena, cells can either aggravate or resolve local immune responses, Sadelain explained. In comparison to chemical drugs, cells can perform multiple tasks: for example, removal, reprogramming or altering macrophages, recruiting immune cells like eosinophils, and giving cues to promote regeneration. He added that cell-based strategies mimic nature's normal process of removing senescent cells through a cellular mechanism.

Nolan underscored the need to search for organizational rules that govern states of pro-resolution or anti-resolution, beyond characterization or description of the state. Given high-level rules, vulnerabilities could be exploited to alter the immune state, he suggested. This process begins at a high level, in examining cellular organizations; subsequently, RNA sequencing or other approaches can be applied to learn more detailed information about the underlying gene networks, for instance. This type of research has made the need for new classes of therapeutics evident. Although cancer has been a useful starting point for understanding wound repair, he highlighted that the CODEX methodology could be used with other models of wound repair or pathology to search for common rules that guide the immune response. These common rules and cellular complexes might elucidate which immune cells are necessary in a certain organization to carry out a particular function, he added.

# 8

# Harnessing the Immune System to Improve Patient Outcomes

---

**Key Points Highlighted by Individual Speakers**

- Convergence of interdisciplinary expertise to leverage tools, models, and approaches could advance discovery and the development of new regenerative immunotherapies. (Botchwey, Elisseeff)
- Heterogeneity—in terms of sex, injury parameters, history of infections, trauma, exposure, and the microbiome, for example—influences the immune state and is important to consider in research and therapeutic development. (Botchwey, Elisseeff)
- To combat health disparities, experimental models could explore the variability of patient outcomes based on ancestry. (Botchwey)
- An area of opportunity in regenerative medicine is developing off-the-shelf cellular therapy products that are cost-effective and accessible to all people who need treatment, wherever they are. (Elisseeff, Schrepfer)
- The complexity of both regenerative medicine products and the immune system presents challenges in predicting the human immune response to therapeutics and in assessing their safety. (Brooks)
- Directing the power of the immune system to improve quality of life is an exciting possibility for patients with autoimmune disorders. (George-Clinton)
- Current research focuses on slowing the progression of pathological fibrosis. Deeper understanding of regenerative mechanisms of the immune system could lead to reversing fibrosis, restoring tissue homeostasis, and even regrowing new organs. (Wynn)

- The approaches of immune evasion and tolerance induction are distinct, and their suitability for a specific patient may depend on the individual's immune status. (Schrepfer)
- To complement strategies of immune evasion and tolerance, approaches to control implanted therapeutic cells, thereby mitigating oncogenic risk, are needed and could be disease-specific or patient-specific. (Schrepfer)
- Academic–industry partnerships could serve an important role to move promising therapies to the clinic. (Elisseeff)
- Using big data and collaborating across disciplines will be important for developing economically feasible, curative, and equitably accessed therapies. (McFarland)

The objective of the sixth and final session of the workshop was to explore areas of clinical therapeutic need amenable to becoming clinical trial candidates. Candidates of particular interest are those that demonstrate proof of principle of a specific therapeutic for clinical indication and that address the immune system's role in improving tissue regeneration. Richard McFarland, chief regulatory officer at the Advanced Regenerative Manufacturing Institute, moderated the session.

## FINAL PANEL DISCUSSION

### Key Challenges and Opportunities for Regenerative Medicine as Offered by the Panelists

To begin the discussion, McFarland noted the aspirational goals of the session, and he asked the panelists to share key challenges and opportunities in their areas of expertise for the field of regenerative medicine. Sherilyn George-Clinton from Multiple Sclerosis: You Are Not Alone remarked that patient communication is both a challenge and an opportunity because low levels of health literacy create space for misunderstanding. At the same time, an opportunity lies in generating better understanding within the patient population, she suggested. Thomas Wynn, vice president of discovery at Pfizer, replied that much of his career has focused on understanding the mechanisms of fibrosis. Attempting to reverse disease and regenerate tissue in a patient with severe fibrosis, and chronic diseases in general, is a major challenge; therefore, one opportunity is developing a deeper understanding of the regenerative mechanisms of the immune system that can be harnessed to address chronic fibrosis, he said. Inflammation resolution is needed to stop the progression of fibrosis, and reversing excess extracellular matrix deposition will require leveraging the immune system, Wynn added. The macrophage may be one of the key cell types in this process due to the ability to produce enzymes that degrade collagen. Wynn expressed his interest in harnessing those mechanisms as an opportunity to reverse fibrosis and restore tissue homeostasis and to better understand how fibrosis impedes regeneration.

A rich area of opportunity lies at the convergence of "domain expertise" in mass spectrometry profiling, metabolomics, and regenerative medicine, said Edward Botchwey, an associate professor in the Department of Biomedical Engineering at the Georgia Institute of Technology. An example of the power of this convergence is the discovery by Charles Serhan, who spoke in an earlier session of the workshop, that bioactive lipids are responsible for active resolution of inflammation. In addition, accessible methods of profiling and modeling injuries could help the field of regenerative engineering effectively leverage endogenous mechanisms of resolution and repair, he suggested. Botchwey and his team have shown through mouse experiments that individual metabolites, such as sphingosine-1-phosphate and leukotriene B4, become elevated at the threshold between muscle injuries that heal successfully and those that yield increased fat and fibrous tissue. Development of effective therapeutic interventions depends on greater understanding of bioactive species and the local mechanisms of their production, degradation, and conversion, said Botchwey. Furthermore, profiling in model systems can improve understanding of the influence of sex, ancestry, and specific injury parameters on repair and regeneration. Perhaps metabolic and immunological signatures could then be used to tailor therapeutics to effectively harness endogenous mechanisms of regeneration, he added.

The key challenge for regenerative medicine and cell therapy is access to medicine, said Sonja Schrepfer, head of the Hypoimmune Platform at Sana Biotechnology. Autologous therapies demonstrate that cell therapy can be effective, and they provide treatment opportunities in both oncology and regenerative medicine. Still, the ability to provide cell therapy to any person, anywhere, at any time is challenging, she said. For instance, specialized allogeneic transplants require overcoming the immunological barrier. However, access to these therapies necessitates distribution of a well-characterized cell product to centers in numerous geographic locations, so off-the-shelf approaches represent a key opportunity, Schrepfer suggested. The ability to provide an off-the-shelf transplant to anyone who needs the therapy will "open the door for regenerative medicine in the future," she added.

The greatest challenge from a preclinical perspective is adequately assessing the safety of regenerative medicine products prior to first-in-human studies, said Danielle Brooks of the Office of Tissues and Advanced Therapies in the U.S. Food and Drug Administration (FDA) Center for Biologics Evaluation and Research. The human immune response to products tested with existing in vitro and in vivo animal models can be difficult to predict. The biggest opportunities in regenerative medicine lie in collaborative workshops, similar to this one hosted by the Forum on Regenerative Medicine, with discussions between disciplines to share novel methods. In addition, early engagement and discussions with the FDA to create multipronged approaches to preclinical development and effectively move products into human trials are helpful and a key opportunity, she said.

The emerging area of initiating immune response by nonmicrobial mechanisms offers great opportunity for discovery, said Jennifer Elisseeff, Morton Goldberg Professor of Ophthalmology and Biomedical Engineering at Johns Hopkins University. Convergence of the fields of autoimmunity, transplants, rejection and tolerance, foreign body response, oncology, and regeneration could lead to complementary discoveries in the immune system. The heterogeneity of patients presents a challenge, but big data could be leveraged to develop immune system therapies that account for the influence of personal history of infections, trauma, exposure, and microbiome on the immune state, Elisseeff said. Biologists, computational scientists, and engineers could work together to build technology to support these efforts, she remarked.

## Patient Perspective on Regenerative Therapeutics

Reflecting on the heterogeneity of patients, George-Clinton said that it is common for members of the multiple sclerosis (MS) community to take prescribed immunomodulators and immunosuppressants. The ability to regenerate nerve cells and myelin cells would be of utmost interest to MS patients. Since many people with MS have multiple autoimmune disorders, the notion that the power of the immune system could be harnessed for good and directed toward improving quality of life is exciting, she added. McFarland emphasized the importance of the patient experience in translating science to cures, noting that scientists can become enthralled with the science and lose sight of the patient experience.

## Possible Roles of Healing and the Immune System in Regenerative Medicine

McFarland asked the panelists about opportunities on the horizon to harness the immune system to improve tissue regeneration and patient experience. Fibrosis has a role in healing; when the body responds to a cut with fibrosis, it prevents harmful bacteria from entering the injury, said Wynn. However, over time fibrosis can be destructive to organs. He and his team are working to slow the progression of harmful fibrosis that impairs organ function, particularly in the lung, muscle, and other tissues. The aim of effectively treating fibrosis can be viewed as three increasingly challenging goals, the first of which involves slowing the progression of the condition, Wynn described. Certain types of fibrosis can be lethal, such as idiopathic pulmonary fibrosis; patients with this progressive disease often die within three to five years of diagnosis. Therefore, slowing the progression of the disease could have significant benefit for patients, he said. A few medicines are able to slow the progression to an extent, but they do not stop it, Wynn noted. The ability to identify the mechanisms driving pathological fibrosis could lead to improvements in slowing its progression. The next goal in treating fibrosis is to reverse scarred tissue; regeneration holds the promise of one day being able to restore normal tissue integrity and architecture. The third objective centers on the ultimate goal of being able to regrow an entirely new organ to replace one that can no longer be repaired. The current focus of therapeutic development is the first stage, slowing progression of fibrosis, said Wynn.

To highlight other promising opportunities, Elisseeff drew an analogy between developments in the cancer immunology field and in regenerative medicine. Initial cancer therapies targeted killing cancer cells, and the field is now working on therapies that use the body's immune system to fight cancer. Similarly, regenerative therapies focused on stem cells and tissue-specific cells, but the field can now also consider methods to create an environment that enables cells to function as intended. For instance, fibrosis can build tissues or it can be pathological; advancements could arise from differentiating those regenerative versus pathological responses, she noted. Although the connection between the immune system and the stroma is currently center stage, the interaction between the immune system and senescence is an exciting area for exploration, added Elisseeff. Finally, academic–industry partnerships could also serve an important role to move promising therapies to the clinic, she said.

Botchwey remarked on the value of converging knowledge and tools from various fields and diverse perspectives, as the Forum on Regenerative Medicine has done with this workshop. Convening is one way to share important advances in manipulating cellular senescence, harnessing the pathways of inflammation resolution, and understanding functional roles and spatial organizations of immune cells and other cell types. He noted current progress in technologies to interpret single-cell data, in ex vivo model systems to control the arrangement of cells in three dimensions, and in engineering biomaterials to present biomolecules to immune cells that alter their function. By bringing these individual areas together more often, new technologies can become more readily available to researchers engaged in discovery, noted Botchwey. Eventually, integration of model systems and approaches can lead to discoveries that otherwise would not have transpired. The virtual world may increase the frequency of such interactions, he added.

## Safety Considerations for Complex Therapeutics

A participant asked how the mechanisms of these complex therapeutic options can be fully understood and how such complicated therapies can meet safety and efficacy guidelines, such as those of the FDA. Botchwey emphasized the importance of good experimental models. For example, mouse injury models have shown that an injury of one size heals, whereas an injury of another size does not, with factors like age and sex controlled. Although the result is not yet completely understood, such models capture as much biological complexity as possible in order to research a question thoroughly. In general, exploration that casts a wide net and involves collaboration with other researchers with valuable expertise may yield new therapeutic discoveries, he said.

McFarland asked Schrepfer to address how the participant's question about safety and efficacy applies to engineering allogeneic donor cells for acceptance by the host immune system. Schrepfer outlined two approaches to encouraging acceptance of transplanted allogeneic cells. The first involves genetically engineering cells to become hypoimmune, meaning that they have been modified to evade recognition by the immune system after transplantation. One benefit of this strategy is that it is stable for the patient, assuming that safe genetic engineering ensures stable cells that will not be recognized by the immune system, she posited. The second approach involves inducing tolerance such that the immune system of the recipient is "educated" to tolerate the transplanted cells. The two approaches are quite different—each involving pros and cons—and the immune status of each individual patient should be considered in determining the best approach, Schrepfer suggested. Considering autoimmune patients as an example, immune evasion may be easier to achieve overall because evasion does not rely on the status of the immune system of the recipient, she said. Both concepts are equally important, and exploring them simultaneously will aid in optimizing methods for cellular transplantation to benefit patients.

Given that transplanted therapeutic cells should be not only shielded from the immune system but also able to replicate, McFarland asked Schrepfer whether there is a risk of oncology carcinogenesis and how risk can be mitigated if the cells are shielded from normal antitumor surveillance. When immune evasion or immune tolerance is in effect, implanted therapeutic cells cannot be controlled using the immune system. Therefore, other methods of controlling cells would be useful, Schrepfer said. Including methods like engineered kill switches, various approaches that are disease specific and possibly patient specific could be developed. This risk is important to consider when creating immune evasion or immune tolerance strategies for allogeneic approaches, and interdisciplinary collaboration and a possible future workshop could help address it, Schrepfer added.

McFarland asked Brooks about nonclinical tools that can improve success in translating approaches from the lab to the clinic. Brooks replied that regenerative medicine products and their responses in human subjects are complex. Rather than make generalized recommendations, the FDA works closely with sponsors from academia and industry to determine the best individual approach for a specific regenerative medicine product. Integrating multiple tools and approaches can help researchers gain a comprehensive view of the product, she said. Researchers may communicate with the FDA early in the development process in order to incorporate feedback into their research efforts, Brooks said. McFarland added that developers could ask themselves questions such as the one that he posed to Schrepfer about carcinogenesis. Asking such questions enables generation of evidence that the FDA uses to inform the benefit–risk assessment conducted with each submission, McFarland said. This approach creates a joint responsibility between the FDA and sponsors to consider not only the potential benefits of regenerative medicine products but also the potential risks. Furthermore, the data produced to answer these questions are likely to support both risk mitigation and the product's benefits, he said. The potential risks to the subject are the FDA's essential concern, and data on what is known and unknown about the response a product will generate in the host environment enable the agency to make the risk–benefit determination, said Brooks. She intends to debrief her team at the FDA on new approaches in use and products shared during the workshop that could potentially enter clinical trials in coming years.

### Emerging Areas in Regenerative Medicine Discussed by Individual Speakers

The field of regenerative medicine requires prolonged focus, said Wynn, noting that after three decades of work on the mechanisms of fibrosis, therapeutics that effectively treat and slow the progression of severe outcomes of fibrotic disease have not been forthcoming. In addition, the emerging area of understanding how the senescence-associated secretory phenotype—referred to as SASP—drives the process of senescence merits attention, he said. Botchwey remarked that interest in the effects of sex on regeneration and aging can be expanded to include consideration of race and health disparities. The fields of immunology and regenerative medicine may engage societal problems—that were brought to the nation's attention again in

2020 by the death of George Floyd—through research that provides insight into the variability of patient outcomes based on ancestry, Botchwey said. Similarly, Elisseeff highlighted the role of sex differences in regenerative medicine, noting that sex differences emerge when examining COVID-19 disease severity and vaccine responses. Genetic associations with certain human leukocyte antigens and the propensity for autoimmune disease should also be considered. In addition, Elisseeff noted her excitement about the potential for the field of regenerative medicine to positively affect patients. To do so, the complex science involved in regenerative therapies might be simplified and translated into manufactured products that can be delivered in a cost effective and impactful way, she said. Lastly, the immune system is often seen as a barrier that must be overcome for a successful transplant, Schrepfer stated, but the immune system holds power that can be utilized to prevent and reverse disease.

### Evolution of the Field of Tissue Regeneration

McFarland concluded the session with a reflection on the evolution of tissue engineering. While completing his Ph.D., McFarland was temporarily distracted from his thesis work by the synopsis of a workshop about tissue engineering (Skalak and Fox, 1988). A professor told him to focus on his thesis, because if the content of the workshop was important, it would still be there after his thesis was complete. Indeed, this area of research is still active three decades later. Even in the early 2000s, as an immunologist and reviewer for the FDA conducting pharmacology and toxicology reviews, the immune system was either deemed a problem or not discussed, he noted. At that time, Carl June, a pioneer in chimeric antigen receptor T-cell therapy, talked about the potential to enhance the capabilities of the immune system using tumor-infiltrating lymphocytes, but the promise was not fully realized. Over 15 years later, Memorial Sloan Kettering and the National Institutes of Health achieved this goal of eliciting a positive immune response. In contrast to earlier approaches that emphasized sterility, current discussion about biocompatibility centers on modifying the environment to be conducive to regeneration of tissues and organs, he said. McFarland concluded by discussing his vision for the future and highlighting the potential for regenerative medicine to have far-reaching positive impact.

## REFLECTIONS ON THE WORKSHOP

Reflections on the workshop's themes were provided by Kimberlee Potter, scientific program manager for the Biomedical Laboratory Research and Development Service at the U.S. Department of Veterans Affairs Office of Research and Development, and Nadya Lumelsky, chief of the Integrative

Biology and Infectious Diseases Branch and director of the Tissue Engineering and Regenerative Medicine Research Program at the National Institute of Dental and Craniofacial Research.

In her concluding remarks, Lumelsky commended the interdisciplinary nature of the workshop and emphasized the value of bringing together the fields of exogenous cell manipulation and endogenous host environment manipulation. The workshop highlighted the emerging view that the immune system has many functions beyond defense from pathogens, as described by Medzhitov, Elisseeff, Moore, and others. Lumelsky emphasized that the absence of inflammation is not the same as inflammation resolution, as Serhan had observed in an earlier session. In fact, many investigators have shown that inflammation suppression can have deleterious effects for tissue regeneration, as optimal resolution of inflammation is critical for tissue regeneration, Lumelsky explained. Throughout the workshop, speakers provided examples of how the immune system could be modulated and its power harnessed to improve patient outcomes (see Box 8-1).

*Tissue or Cell-based Transplantation and Exogenous Manipulation of Donor Cells*

Presenting lessons from organ transplant immunology that might apply to regenerative medicine, Sykes outlined different transplantation protocols, efforts to move toward immune tolerance, and how various techniques access different immune mechanisms. By reducing the need for immunosuppressive drugs and therefore the devastating side effects they can cause, induction of immune tolerance could prove beneficial to patients because they can alleviate injection concerns as well as leave the immune system intact to combat infections, Potter summarized. Adding to the discussion, Schrepfer, Le Blanc, and Valamehr shared various strategies to evade immune detection or induce immune tolerance in the host to increase acceptance of exogenous cell therapies. Finally, Sadelain discussed anti-cancer CAR T immunotherapies featuring engineered T cells, which he described as "living drugs." Lumelsky reiterated that CAR T therapies may be a future tool for removing senescent cells and modulating tissue regeneration.

*Endogenous Mechanisms of Repair and their Modulation*

The workshop also featured approaches that do not require exogenous cell injection; rather, the strategies manipulate endogenous modulators of cell processes to repair or build new tissue, Lumelsky summarized. For example, Blau discussed the activity of prostaglandin E2, an inflammatory mediator, in augmenting skeletal muscle and preventing sarcopenia, an age-related muscle wasting condition. Hajishengallis shared how a secreted

> **BOX 8-1**
> **Ideas about the Future of Regenerative Medicine with Regard to the Immune System as Shared by Individual Presenters**
>
> **Convergence across Fields**
> - Integrative, multidisciplinary approaches could accelerate scientific discovery and hold therapeutic potential. (Botchwey, Elisseeff, Kirkland, Sadtler)
> - Combining different modalities for niche manipulation could be a powerful strategy to promote tissue regeneration. (Blau, Hajishengallis, Moore)
> - Future therapies could leverage strategies to both promote tissue repair and remove factors that inhibit repair. (Botchwey, Elisseeff, Medzhitov, Serhan)
>
> **Spatiotemporal Modulation and Customized Therapies**
> - Targeted therapies require customization based on features like tissue type, timing of intervention, patient profile, and more. (Hajishengallis, Jenq)
> - Optimal timing for treatment intervention varies across organs and tissues and should be developed for each system or application. (Elisseeff, Moore, Serhan)
> - Modulation can include both local and systemic strategies, which influence one another. (Elisseeff, Medzhitov)
>
> **Potential Therapeutic Advances**
> - Strategies to achieve immune tolerance and evasion would obviate the need for immunosuppressive drugs with negative side effects and, thereby, benefit patients. (Schrepfer, Sykes, Valamehr)
> - Senolytics target senescent cells rather than a single molecule or pathway. The combination of senolytics and antifibrotic agents can have a synergistic, pro-healing effect. (Kirkland)

protein called DEL-1 promotes inflammation resolution and tissue regeneration in periodontitis. Lumelsky also highlighted the importance of inflammation resolution and the pro-resolving mediators that Serhan pioneered.

Several of these key mediators exhibit altered expression in aging, and the role of senescent cells in disease and aging was discussed by Kirkland. He explained that aging involves interrelated fundamental processes, and interventions that target one process tend to also affect other processes of aging. Thus, senolytic agents could possibly affect pleiotropic aging in various directions, preventing and delaying age-related conditions and diseases, Lumelsky summarized. Lumelsky expressed her hope that someday many conditions will be amenable to therapies that manipulate endogenous modulators of cell regeneration, cell degeneration, and aging and that exogenous cell injection may no longer be necessary for building new tissues.

- Novel pro-resolving mediators shorten the inflammation resolution interval and can promote tissue repair. (Serhan)
- Chimeric antigen receptor (CAR) T-cell therapies use engineered T cells as "living drugs" and represent a potential tool for treating many pathologies. (Sadelain)

**Tools and Methods to Better Understand the Immune System**
- Biomaterials can be used to model the immune microenvironment and understand the immune response in disease and wound healing as well as modulate the environment to optimize healing. (Elisseeff, Moore, Sadtler)
- CODEX is a multiplexing imaging tool, and the imaging data can be used to extrapolate dynamic behavior and cellular relationships. (Nolan)
- Big data and computational tools can be used to map the immune environment. (Elisseeff, Nolan, Sadtler)

**Recognizing and Harnessing the Potential of the Immune System**
- The immune system is often seen as a barrier, but its power can be leveraged to prevent or reverse disease. (McFarland, Sadelain, Schrepfer, Wynn)
- Harnessing the power of the immune system to benefit patients and improve their quality of life is an exciting possibility for patients. (George-Clinton)
- The field would benefit from iterative hypothesis generation, moving from bench to bedside and back to bench. (Jenq, Sadtler)
- Off-the-shelf strategies are a promising avenue to promote equitable access to medicines for patients who need them, no matter where they live. (Elisseeff, Schrepfer, Valamehr)

NOTE: These points were made by the individual workshop speakers and participants identified above. They are not intended to reflect a consensus among workshop participants.

*Tools to Investigate and Modulate the Immune System*

The workshop also included examples of tools and concepts to monitor, investigate, and optimize the immune environment. For instance, Medzhitov introduced concepts of tissue homeostasis and division of labor among different cell types. These concepts could serve as models for ideas being developed in tissue regeneration, suggested Potter. Moreover, systems biology approaches may enable researchers to better understand the complexities of biological tissues. Nolan provided an overview of the multiplexing imaging tool CODEX and how the data from it can be used to define cellular neighborhoods. Nolan emphasized the importance of interfaces between cellular neighborhoods, and results indicate that the local biology of these neighborhoods may have prognostic value for diagnosis and clinical treatment. Nolan's concept of cellular neighborhoods resonates with Medzhitov's discussion of the functional and structural role of cellular units within tissues, Lumelsky noted.

Biomaterials can be used to model the immune microenvironment to better understand the immune response in disease and wound healing, as presented by Moore, Elisseeff, and Sadtler. Using biomaterials, Moore and her team modeled immune cell mediation in wound healing and profiled the B-cell responses to better understand variability in wound healing. Elisseeff described the tissue microenvironment as an intervention target and highlighted the growing role of big data in this period of discovery. The development of biomaterials with intentionally designed functions may enable researchers and physicians to encourage desired immune responses, Lumelsky summarized. Sadtler had also said that rational design for creating anti-fibrotic and pro-healing biomaterials depends on understanding the fundamental biology. Given their ability to activate biomolecules, these biomaterials could be especially useful; furthermore, the capacity to modulate spatiotemporal components of the niche could augment the effectiveness of these biomaterials, Lumelsky commented.

*Imagining the Future of Regenerative Medicine*

Reiterating an idea proposed by Jenq, who described how variability in human data can be used to generate new hypotheses, Potter emphasized the importance of reverse engineering hypotheses. Sadtler also highlighted the potential value of integrative, iterative approaches that apply preclinical and quantitative modeling data to clinical therapeutics. Iterative hypothesis generation that incorporates "going from bench to bedside and back to bench" has potential to benefit patients while also enriching foundational knowledge about the role of the immune system in improving tissue regeneration, Lumelsky reflected.

Lumelsky said that the integration of different modalities and therapies emerged as a theme throughout the interdisciplinary workshop, summarizing points made by Kirkland, Elisseeff, Botchwey, and others (see Box 8-1). Future immunotherapies will likely include combination therapies that promote tissue regeneration while inhibiting fibrosis, she said. Combining regenerative medicine, immunology, and biomaterial design, the field of regenerative immunology has the potential to both promote endogenous tissue regeneration and affect the survival and regeneration of exogenous cell-based therapies, Lumelsky remarked in response to Elisseeff's work.

## Final Thoughts

Despite the challenges presented by the immune system, the many scientific and therapeutic opportunities for regenerative medicine are exciting and could benefit patients in the near future; indeed, "all challenges are connected to an opportunity," Elisseeff said. The field of regenerative medicine is evolving, and new regenerative immunotherapies can be created through interdisciplinary collaboration to further the goal of helping patients, she said. In this era, big data and collaboration across sciences will be important in achieving the creation of economically feasible, curative therapies that can be distributed to diverse populations, said McFarland. He added that this can be carried out in a way that decreases the disparity that has been inherent in clinical services. Importantly, this field offers the opportunity of moving beyond treatments to cures, McFarland said.

# References

Adler, M., A. Mayo, X. Zhou, R. A. Franklin, J. B. Jacox, R. Medzhitov, and U. Alon. 2018. Endocytosis as a stabilizing mechanism for tissue homeostasis. *Proceedings of the National Academy of Sciences of the United States of America* 115(8):E1926–E1935.

Amor, C., J. Feucht, J. Leibold, Y. J. Ho, C. Zhu, D. Alonso-Curbelo, J. Mansilla-Soto, J. A. Boyer, X. Li, T. Giavridis, A. Kulick, S. Houlihan, E. Peerschke, S. L. Friedman, V. Ponomarev, A. Piersigilli, M. Sadelain, and S. W. Lowe. 2020. Senolytic CAR T cells reverse senescence-associated pathologies. *Nature* 583(7814):127–132.

Anderson, J. M., A. Rodriguez, and D. T. Chang. 2008. Foreign body reaction to biomaterials. *Seminars in Immunology* 20(2):86–100.

Arnardottir, H. H., J. Dalli, R. A. Colas, M. Shinohara, and C. N. Serhan. 2014. Aging delays resolution of acute inflammation in mice: Reprogramming the host response with novel nano-proresolving medicines. *Journal of Immunology* 193(8):4235–4244.

Badylak, S. F., J. E. Valentin, A. K. Ravindra, G. P. McCabe, and A. M. Stewart-Akers. 2008. Macrophage phenotype as a determinant of biologic scaffold remodeling. *Tissue Engineering Part A* 14(11):1835–1842.

Bellantuono, I. 2018. Find drugs that delay many diseases of old age. *Nature* 554(7692):293–295.

Bemelman, F., K. Honey, E. Adams, S. Cobbold, and H. Waldmann. 1998. Bone marrow transplantation induces either clonal deletion or infectious tolerance depending on the dose. *Journal of Immunology* 160(6):2645–2648.

Bhate, S. S., G. L. Barlow, C. M. Schürch, and G. P. Nolan. 2021. Tissue schematics map the specialization of immune tissue motifs and their appropriation by tumors. *Cell Systems*.

Bigenzahn, S., P. Blaha, Z. Koporc, I. Pree, E. Selzer, H. Bergmeister, F. Wrba, C. Heusser, K. Wagner, F. Muehlbacher, and T. Wekerle. 2005. The role of non-deletional tolerance mechanisms in a murine model of mixed chimerism with costimulation blockade. *American Journal of Transplantation* 5(6):1237–1247.

Blau, H. M., B. D. Cosgrove, and A. T. Ho. 2015. The central role of muscle stem cells in regenerative failure with aging. *Nature Medicine* 21(8):854–862.

Boberg, E., L. von Bahr, G. Afram, C. Lindstrom, P. Ljungman, N. Heldring, P. Petzelbauer, K. Garming Legert, N. Kadri, and K. Le Blanc. 2020. Treatment of chronic GVHD with mesenchymal stromal cells induces durable responses: A phase II study. *Stem Cells Translational Medicine* 9(10):1190–1202.

Botelho, J., V. Machado, Y. Leira, L. Proenca, L. Chambrone, and J. J. Mendes. 2021. Economic burden of periodontitis in the United States and Europe—An updated estimation. *Journal of Periodontology*: 1-7.

Brentjens, R. J., M. L. Davila, I. Riviere, J. Park, X. Wang, L. G. Cowell, S. Bartido, J. Stefanski, C. Taylor, M. Olszewska, O. Borquez-Ojeda, J. Qu, T. Wasielewska, Q. He, Y. Bernal, I. V. Rijo, C. Hedvat, R. Kobos, K. Curran, P. Steinherz, J. Jurcic, T. Rosenblat, P. Maslak, M. Frattini, and M. Sadelain. 2013. CD19-targeted T cells rapidly induce molecular remissions in adults with chemotherapy-refractory acute lymphoblastic leukemia. *Science Translational Medicine* 5(177):177ra138.

Brentjens, R. J., J.-B. Latouche, E. Santos, F. Marti, M. C. Gong, C. Lyddane, P. D. King, S. Larson, M. Weiss, I. Rivière, and M. Sadelain. 2003. Eradication of systemic B-cell tumors by genetically targeted human T lymphocytes co-stimulated by CD80 and interleukin-15. *Nature Medicine* 9(3):279–286.

Browne, S., and A. Pandit. 2015. Biomaterial-mediated modification of the local inflammatory environment. *Frontiers in Bioengineering and Biotechnology* 3(67):67.

Burns, E. R., J. A. Stevens, and R. Lee. 2016. The direct costs of fatal and non-fatal falls among older adults—United States. *Journal of Safety Research* 58:99–103.

Chen, X., L. Poncette, and T. Blankenstein. 2017. Human TCR-MHC coevolution after divergence from mice includes increased nontemplate-encoded CDR3 diversity. *Journal of Experimental Medicine* 214(11):3417–3433.

Cheng, A., C. E. Vantucci, L. Krishnan, M. A. Ruehle, T. Kotanchek, L. B. Wood, K. Roy, and R. E. Guldberg. 2021. Early systemic immune biomarkers predict bone regeneration after trauma. *Proceedings of the National Academy of Sciences of the United States of America* 118(8).

Cherry, C., D. R. Maestas, J. Han, J. I. Andorko, P. Cahan, E. J. Fertig, L. X. Garmire, and J. H. Elisseeff. 2021. Computational reconstruction of the signalling networks surrounding implanted biomaterials from single-cell transcriptomics. *Nature Biomedical Engineering* 5(10):1228–1238.

Chiang, N., X. de la Rosa, S. Libreros, H. Pan, J. M. Dreyfuss, and C. N. Serhan. 2021. Cysteinyl-specialized proresolving mediators link resolution of infectious inflammation and tissue regeneration via TRAF3 activation. *Proceedings of the National Academy of Sciences of the United States of America* 118(10):e2013374118.

Chiurchiu, V., A. Leuti, J. Dalli, A. Jacobsson, L. Battistini, M. Maccarrone, and C. N. Serhan. 2016. Proresolving lipid mediators resolvin D1, resolvin D2, and maresin 1 are critical in modulating T cell responses. *Science Translational Medicine* 8(353):353ra111.

Choi, E. Y., E. Chavakis, M. A. Czabanka, H. F. Langer, L. Fraemohs, M. Economopoulou, R. K. Kundu, A. Orlandi, Y. Y. Zheng, D. A. Prieto, C. M. Ballantyne, S. L. Constant, W. C. Aird, T. Papayannopoulou, C. G. Gahmberg, M. C. Udey, P. Vajkoczy, T. Quertermous, S. Dimmeler, C. Weber, and T. Chavakis. 2008. Del-1, an endogenous leukocyte-endothelial adhesion inhibitor, limits inflammatory cell recruitment. *Science* 322(5904):1101–1104.

Choi, E. Y., J. H. Lim, A. Neuwirth, M. Economopoulou, A. Chatzigeorgiou, K. J. Chung, S. Bittner, S. H. Lee, H. Langer, M. Samus, H. Kim, G. S. Cho, T. Ziemssen, K. Bdeir, E. Chavakis, J. Y. Koh, L. Boon, K. Hosur, S. R. Bornstein, S. G. Meuth, G. Hajishengallis, and T. Chavakis. 2015. Developmental endothelial locus-1 is a homeostatic factor in the central nervous system limiting neuroinflammation and demyelination. *Molecular Psychiatry* 20(7):880–888.

Chung, L., D. R. Maestas, Jr., A. Lebid, A. Mageau, G. D. Rosson, X. Wu, M. T. Wolf, A. J. Tam, I. Vanderzee, X. Wang, J. I. Andorko, H. Zhang, R. Narain, K. Sadtler, H. Fan, D. Cihakova, C. J. Le Saux, F. Housseau, D. M. Pardoll, and J. H. Elisseeff. 2020. Interleukin 17 and senescent cells regulate the foreign body response to synthetic material implants in mice and humans. *Science Translational Medicine* 12(539):eaax3799.

Cianci, E., A. Recchiuti, O. Trubiani, F. Diomede, M. Marchisio, S. Miscia, R. A. Colas, J. Dalli, C. N. Serhan, and M. Romano. 2016. Human periodontal stem cells release specialized proresolving mediators and carry immunomodulatory and prohealing properties regulated by lipoxins. *Stem Cells Translational Medicine* 5(1):20–32.

Couzin-Frankel, J. 2013. Breakthrough of the year 2013. Cancer immunotherapy. *Science* 342(6165):1432–1433.

Dalli, J., N. Chiang, and C. N. Serhan. 2014. Identification of 14-series sulfido-conjugated mediators that promote resolution of infection and organ protection. *Proceedings of the National Academy of Sciences of the United States of America* 111(44):E4753–4761.

de la Rosa, X., P. C. Norris, N. Chiang, A. R. Rodriguez, B. W. Spur, and C. N. Serhan. 2018. Identification and complete stereochemical assignments of the new resolvin conjugates in tissue regeneration in human tissues that stimulate proresolving phagocyte functions and tissue regeneration. *American Journal of Pathology* 188(4):950–966.

de Witte, S. F. H., A. M. Merino, M. Franquesa, T. Strini, J. A. A. van Zoggel, S. S. Korevaar, F. Luk, M. Gargesha, L. O'Flynn, D. Roy, S. J. Elliman, P. N. Newsome, C. C. Baan, and M. J. Hoogduijn. 2017. Cytokine treatment optimises the immunotherapeutic effects of umbilical cord-derived MSC for treatment of inflammatory liver disease. *Stem Cell Research & Therapy* 8(1):140.

Deuse, T., X. Hu, S. Agbor-Enoh, M. K. Jang, M. Alawi, C. Saygi, A. Gravina, G. Tediashvili, V. Q. Nguyen, Y. Liu, H. Valantine, L. L. Lanier, and S. Schrepfer. 2021a. The SIRP – CD47 immune checkpoint in NK cells. *Journal of Experimental Medicine* 218(3).

Deuse, T., X. Hu, S. Agbor-Enoh, M. Koch, M. H. Spitzer, A. Gravina, M. Alawi, A. Marishta, B. Peters, Z. Kosaloglu-Yalcin, Y. Yang, R. Rajalingam, D. Wang, B. Nashan, R. Kiefmann, H. Reichenspurner, H. Valantine, I. L. Weissman, and S. Schrepfer. 2019. De novo mutations in mitochondrial DNA of iPSCs produce immunogenic neoepitopes in mice and humans. *Nature Biotechnology* 37(10):1137–1144.

Deuse, T., G. Tediashvili, X. Hu, A. Gravina, A. Tamenang, D. Wang, A. Connolly, C. Mueller, B. Mallavia, M. R. Looney, M. Alawi, L. L. Lanier, and S. Schrepfer. 2021b. Hypoimmune induced pluripotent stem cell-derived cell therapeutics treat cardiovascular and pulmonary diseases in immunocompetent allogeneic mice. *Proceedings of the National Academy of Sciences of the United States of America* 118(28).

Deuse, T., D. Wang, M. Stubbendorff, R. Itagaki, A. Grabosch, L. C. Greaves, M. Alawi, A. Grunewald, X. Hu, X. Hua, J. Velden, H. Reichenspurner, R. C. Robbins, R. Jaenisch, I. L. Weissman, and S. Schrepfer. 2015. SCNT-derived ESCs with mismatched mitochondria trigger an immune response in allogeneic hosts. *Cell Stem Cell* 16(1):33–38.

Doloff, J. C., O. Veiseh, A. J. Vegas, H. H. Tam, S. Farah, M. Ma, J. Li, A. Bader, A. Chiu, A. Sadraei, S. Aresta-Dasilva, M. Griffin, S. Jhunjhunwala, M. Webber, S. Siebert, K. Tang, M. Chen, E. Langan, N. Dholokia, R. Thakrar, M. Qi, J. Oberholzer, D. L. Greiner, R. Langer, and D. G. Anderson. 2017. Colony stimulating factor-1 receptor is a central component of the foreign body response to biomaterial implants in rodents and non-human primates. *Nature Materials* 16(6):671–680.

Domenig, C., A. Sanchez-Fueyo, J. Kurtz, S. P. Alexopoulos, C. Mariat, M. Sykes, T. B. Strom, and X. X. Zheng. 2005. Roles of deletion and regulation in creating mixed chimerism and allograft tolerance using a nonlymphoablative irradiation-free protocol. *Journal of Immunology* 175(1):51–60.

Dort, J., Z. Orfi, P. Fabre, T. Molina, T. C. Conte, K. Greffard, O. Pellerito, J. F. Bilodeau, and N. A. Dumont. 2021. Resolvin-D2 targets myogenic cells and improves muscle regeneration in Duchenne muscular dystrophy. *Nature Communications* 12(1):6264.

Duran-Struuck, R., H. P. Sondermeijer, L. Buhler, P. Alonso-Guallart, J. Zitsman, Y. Kato, A. Wu, A. N. McMurchy, D. Woodland, A. Griesemer, M. Martinez, S. Boskovic, T. Kawai, A. B. Cosimi, Y. G. Yang, Z. Hu, C. S. Wuu, A. Slate, M. Mapara, S. Baker, R. Tokarz, V. D'Agati, S. Hammer, M. Pereira, W. I. Lipkin, T. Wekerle, M. Levings, and M. Sykes. 2017. Effect of ex vivo-expanded recipient regulatory T cells on hematopoietic chimerism and kidney allograft tolerance across MHC barriers in cynomolgus macaques. *Transplantation* 101(2):274–283.

Eskan, M. A., R. Jotwani, T. Abe, J. Chmelar, J. H. Lim, S. Liang, P. A. Ciero, J. L. Krauss, F. Li, M. Rauner, L. C. Hofbauer, E. Y. Choi, K. J. Chung, A. Hashim, M. A. Curtis, T. Chavakis, and G. Hajishengallis. 2012. The leukocyte integrin antagonist Del-1 inhibits IL-17-mediated inflammatory bone loss. *Nature Immunology* 13(5):465–473.

Faust, H. J., H. Zhang, J. Han, M. T. Wolf, O. H. Jeon, K. Sadtler, A. N. Pena, L. Chung, D. R. Maestas, Jr., A. J. Tam, D. M. Pardoll, J. Campisi, F. Housseau, D. Zhou, C. O. Bingham, 3rd, and J. H. Elisseeff. 2020. IL-17 and immunologically induced senescence regulate response to injury in osteoarthritis. *Journal of Clinical Investigation* 130(10):5493–5507.

Fehr, T., F. Haspot, J. Mollov, M. Chittenden, T. Hogan, and M. Sykes. 2008. Alloreactive CD8 T cell tolerance requires recipient B cells, dendritic cells, and MHC class II. *Journal of Immunology* 181(1):165–173.

Fehr, T., C. L. Lucas, J. Kurtz, T. Onoe, G. Zhao, T. Hogan, C. Vallot, A. Rao, and M. Sykes. 2010. A CD8 T cell–intrinsic role for the calcineurin-NFAT pathway for tolerance induction in vivo. *Blood* 115(6):1280–1287.

Fehr, T., Y. Takeuchi, J. Kurtz, T. Wekerle, and M. Sykes. 2005. Early regulation of CD8 T cell alloreactivity by $CD4^+CD25^-$ T cells in recipients of anti-CD154 antibody and allogeneic BMT is followed by rapid peripheral deletion of donor-reactive $CD8^+$ T cells, precluding a role for sustained regulation. *European Journal of Immunology* 35(9):2679–2690.

Galleu, A., Y. Riffo-Vasquez, C. Trento, C. Lomas, L. Dolcetti, T. S. Cheung, M. von Bonin, L. Barbieri, K. Halai, S. Ward, L. Weng, R. Chakraverty, G. Lombardi, F. M. Watt, K. Orchard, D. I. Marks, J. Apperley, M. Bornhauser, H. Walczak, C. Bennett, and F. Dazzi. 2017. Apoptosis in mesenchymal stromal cells induces in vivo recipient–mediated immunomodulation. *Science Translational Medicine* 9(416).

Gaudilliere, B., G. K. Fragiadakis, R. V. Bruggner, M. Nicolau, R. Finck, M. Tingle, J. Silva, E. A. Ganio, C. G. Yeh, W. J. Maloney, J. I. Huddleston, S. B. Goodman, M. M. Davis, S. C. Bendall, W. J. Fantl, M. S. Angst, and G. P. Nolan. 2014. Clinical recovery from surgery correlates with single-cell immune signatures. *Science Translational Medicine* 6(255):255ra131.

Gavin, C., E. Boberg, L. Von Bahr, M. Bottai, A. T. Andren, A. Wernerson, L. C. Davies, R. V. Sugars, and K. Le Blanc. 2019a. Tissue immune profiles supporting response to mesenchymal stromal cell therapy in acute graft-versus-host disease-a gut feeling. *Stem Cell Research & Therapy* 10(1):334.

Gavin, C., S. Meinke, N. Heldring, K. A. Heck, A. Achour, E. Iacobaeus, P. Hoglund, K. Le Blanc, and N. Kadri. 2019b. The complement system is essential for the phagocytosis of mesenchymal stromal cells by monocytes. *Frontiers in Immunology* 10:2249.

Globerson Levin, A., I. Riviere, Z. Eshhar, and M. Sadelain. 2021. CAR T cells: Building on the CD19 paradigm. *European Journal of Immunology* 51(9):2151–2163.

Goltsev, Y., N. Samusik, J. Kennedy-Darling, S. Bhate, M. Hale, G. Vazquez, S. Black, and G. P. Nolan. 2018. Deep profiling of mouse splenic architecture with CODEX multiplexed imaging. *Cell* 174(4):968–981 e915.

Goncalves, F. D. C., F. Luk, S. S. Korevaar, R. Bouzid, A. H. Paz, C. Lopez-Iglesias, C. C. Baan, A. Merino, and M. J. Hoogduijn. 2017. Membrane particles generated from mesenchymal stromal cells modulate immune responses by selective targeting of pro-inflammatory monocytes. *Scientific Reports* 7(1):12100.

Gregoire, C., C. Ritacco, M. Hannon, L. Seidel, L. Delens, L. Belle, S. Dubois, S. Veriter, C. Lechanteur, A. Briquet, S. Servais, G. Ehx, Y. Beguin, and F. Baron. 2019. Comparison of mesenchymal stromal cells from different origins for the treatment of graft-vs.-host-disease in a humanized mouse model. *Frontiers in Immunology* 10:619.

Hachim, D., S. T. Lopresti, C. C. Yates, and B. N. Brown. 2017. Shifts in macrophage phenotype at the biomaterial interface via IL-4 eluting coatings are associated with improved implant integration. *Biomaterials* 112:95–107.

Hajishengallis, G., and T. Chavakis. 2021. Local and systemic mechanisms linking periodontal disease and inflammatory comorbidities. *Nature Reviews Immunology* 21(7):426–440.

Han, J., C. Cherry, A. Ruta, D. R. Maestas, J. C. Mejias, H. H. Nguyen, E. J. Fertig, F. Housseau, S. Ganguly, E. M. Moore, A. J. Tam, D. M. Pardoll, and J. H. Elisseeff. 2021 (unpublished). *Age-related immune-stromal networks inhibit response to regenerative immunotherapies*. Cold Spring Harbor, NY: Cold Spring Harbor Laboratory.

Haspot, F., T. Fehr, C. Gibbons, G. Zhao, T. Hogan, T. Honjo, G. J. Freeman, and M. Sykes. 2008. Peripheral deletional tolerance of alloreactive CD8 but not CD4 T cells is dependent on the PD-1/PD-L1 pathway. *Blood* 112(5):2149–2155.

Hasturk, H., G. Hajishengallis, Forsyth Institute Center for Translational Research staff, J. D. Lambris, D. C. Mastellos, and D. Yancopoulou. 2021. Phase IIa clinical trial of complement C3 inhibitor AMY-101 in adults with periodontal inflammation. *Journal of Clinical Investigation* 131(23).

Hayase, E., T. Hayase, C.-C. Chang, T. Miyama, J. L. Karmouch, W.-B. Tsai, M. A. Jamal, and R. R. Jenq. 2021. Carbapenem antibiotics promote mucus degradation by bacteroides and aggravate graft-versus-host disease. *Blood* 138(Supplement 1):85–85.

Heredia, J. E., L. Mukundan, F. M. Chen, A. A. Mueller, R. C. Deo, R. M. Locksley, T. A. Rando, and A. Chawla. 2013. Type 2 innate signals stimulate fibro/adipogenic progenitors to facilitate muscle regeneration. *Cell* 153(2):376–388.

Hickey, J. W., E. K. Neumann, A. J. Radtke, J. M. Camarillo, R. T. Beuschel, A. Albanese, E. McDonough, J. Hatler, A. E. Wiblin, J. Fisher, J. Croteau, E. C. Small, A. Sood, R. M. Caprioli, R. M. Angelo, G. P. Nolan, K. Chung, S. M. Hewitt, R. N. Germain, J. M. Spraggins, E. Lundberg, M. P. Snyder, N. L. Kelleher, and S. K. Saka. 2021. Spatial mapping of protein composition and tissue organization: A primer for multiplexed antibody-based imaging. *Nature Methods*: 1-12.

Hickson, L. J., L. G. P. Langhi Prata, S. A. Bobart, T. K. Evans, N. Giorgadze, S. K. Hashmi, S. M. Herrmann, M. D. Jensen, Q. Jia, K. L. Jordan, T. A. Kellogg, S. Khosla, D. M. Koerber, A. B. Lagnado, D. K. Lawson, N. K. Lebrasseur, L. O. Lerman, K. M. McDonald, T. J. McKenzie, J. F. Passos, R. J. Pignolo, T. Pirtskhalava, I. M. Saadiq, K. K. Schaefer, S. C. Textor, S. G. Victorelli, T. L. Volkman, A. Xue, M. A. Wentworth, E. O. Wissler Gerdes, Y. Zhu, T. Tchkonia, and J. L. Kirkland. 2019. Senolytics decrease senescent cells in humans: Preliminary report from a clinical trial of dasatinib plus quercetin in individuals with diabetic kidney disease. *EBioMedicine* 47:446–456.

Hillel, A. T., S. Unterman, Z. Nahas, B. Reid, J. M. Coburn, J. Axelman, J. J. Chae, Q. Guo, R. Trow, A. Thomas, Z. Hou, S. Lichtsteiner, D. Sutton, C. Matheson, P. Walker, N. David, S. Mori, J. M. Taube, and J. H. Elisseeff. 2011. Photoactivated composite biomaterial for soft tissue restoration in rodents and in humans. *Science Translational Medicine* 3(93):93ra67.

Ho, A. T. V., A. R. Palla, M. R. Blake, N. D. Yucel, Y. X. Wang, K. E. G. Magnusson, C. A. Holbrook, P. E. Kraft, S. L. Delp, and H. M. Blau. 2017. Prostaglandin E2 is essential for efficacious skeletal muscle stem-cell function, augmenting regeneration and strength. *Proceedings of the National Academy of Sciences of the United States of America* 114(26):6675–6684.

Ho, Y. T., T. Shimbo, E. Wijaya, Y. Ouchi, E. Takaki, R. Yamamoto, Y. Kikuchi, Y. Kaneda, and K. Tamai. 2018. Chromatin accessibility identifies diversity in mesenchymal stem cells from different tissue origins. *Scientific Reports* 8(1):17765.

Hollyman, D., J. Stefanski, M. Przybylowski, S. Bartido, O. Borquez-Ojeda, C. Taylor, R. Yeh, V. Capacio, M. Olszewska, J. Hosey, M. Sadelain, R. J. Brentjens, and I. Riviere. 2009. Manufacturing validation of biologically functional T cells targeted to CD19 antigen for autologous adoptive cell therapy. *Journal of Immunotherapy* 32(2):169–180.

Hu, X., M. Dao, K. White, R. Clarke, S. Landry, R. Basco, C. Gattis, E. Tham, E. Luo, A. Tucker, C. Bandoro, E. Chu, J. Kim, C. Young, W. E. Dowdle, E. J. Rebar, T. J. Fry, and S. Schrepfer. 2021. Abstract LB144: Overexpression of CD47 protects hypoimmune CAR T cells from innate immune cell killing. *Cancer Research* 81(13 Supplement):LB144.

Hunt, D., D. W. Chapa, B. Hess, K. Swanick, and A. Hovanec. 2015. The importance of resistance training in the treatment of sarcopenia. *Journal of Nursing Education and Practice* 5(3):39–43. doi: 10.5430/jnep.v5n3p39.

Iske, J., M. Seyda, T. Heinbokel, R. Maenosono, K. Minami, Y. Nian, M. Quante, C. S. Falk, H. Azuma, F. Martin, J. F. Passos, C. U. Niemann, T. Tchkonia, J. L. Kirkland, A. Elkhal, and S. G. Tullius. 2020. Senolytics prevent mt-DNA-induced inflammation and promote the survival of aged organs following transplantation. *Nature Commununications* 11(1):4289.

Iwata, Y., A. Yoshizaki, K. Komura, K. Shimizu, F. Ogawa, T. Hara, E. Muroi, S. Bae, M. Takenaka, T. Yukami, M. Hasegawa, M. Fujimoto, Y. Tomita, T. F. Tedder, and S. Sato. 2009. CD19, a response regulator of B lymphocytes, regulates wound healing through hyaluronan-induced TLR4 signaling. *American Journal of Pathology* 175(2):649–660.

Jagasia, M., A. Lazaryan, C. R. Bachier, A. Salhotra, D. J. Weisdorf, B. Zoghi, J. Essell, L. Green, O. Schueller, J. Patel, A. Zanin-Zhorov, J. M. Weiss, Z. Yang, D. Eiznhamer, S. K. Aggarwal, B. R. Blazar, and S. J. Lee. 2021. ROCK2 inhibition with belumosudil (KD025) for the treatment of chronic graft-versus-host disease. *Journal of Clinical Oncology* 39(17):1888–1898.

Janeway, C. A., P. Travers, M. Walport, and M. Shlomchik. 2001. *Immunobiology: The immune system in health and disease*, 5th ed. New York: Garland Science.

Jenq, R. R., and M. R. van den Brink. 2010. Allogeneic haematopoietic stem cell transplantation: Individualized stem cell and immune therapy of cancer. *Nature Reviews Cancer* 10(3):213–221.

Jing, Y., Z. Ni, J. Wu, L. Higgins, T. W. Markowski, D. S. Kaufman, and B. Walcheck. 2015. Identification of an ADAM17 cleavage region in human CD16 (Fc RIII) and the engineering of a non-cleavable version of the receptor in NK cells. *PLOS ONE* 10(3):e0121788.

Jones, J. M., R. Wilson, and P. M. Bealmear. 1971. Mortality and gross pathology of secondary disease in germfree mouse radiation chimeras. *Radiation Research* 45(3):577–588.

Julier, Z., A. J. Park, P. S. Briquez, and M. M. Martino. 2017. Promoting tissue regeneration by modulating the immune system. *Acta Biomaterialia* 53:13–28.

Jun, J. I., and L. F. Lau. 2011. Taking aim at the extracellular matrix: CCN proteins as emerging therapeutic targets. *Nature Reviews Drug Discovery* 10(12):945-963.

June, C. H., and M. Sadelain. 2018. Chimeric antigen receptor therapy. *The New England Journal of Medicine* 379(1):64–73.

Kasikis, S., J. Baez, I. Gandhi, S. Grupp, C. L. Kitko, S. Kowalyk, P. Merli, G. Morales, M. A. Pulsipher, M. Qayed, M. Wolfl, G. Yanik, F. See, J. Hayes, F. Grossman, E. Burke, R. Young, J. E. Levine, and J. L. M. Ferrara. 2021. Mesenchymal stromal cell therapy induces high responses and survival in children with steroid refractory GVHD and poor risk biomarkers. *Bone Marrow Transplantation* 56(11):2869–2870.

Kasler, H., and E. Verdin. 2021. How inflammaging diminishes adaptive immunity. *Nature Aging* 1(1):24–25.

Kassebaum, N. J., E. Bernabe, M. Dahiya, B. Bhandari, C. J. Murray, and W. Marcenes. 2014. Global burden of severe periodontitis in 1990–2010: A systematic review and meta-regression. *Journal of Dental Research* 93(11):1045–1053.

Kawai, T., A. B. Cosimi, T. R. Spitzer, N. Tolkoff-Rubin, M. Suthanthiran, S. L. Saidman, J. Shaffer, F. I. Preffer, R. Ding, V. Sharma, J. A. Fishman, B. Dey, D. S. C. Ko, M. Hertl, N. B. Goes, W. Wong, W. W. Williams, Jr., R. B. Colvin, M. Sykes, and D. H. Sachs. 2008. HLA-mismatched renal transplantation without maintenance immunosuppression. *The New England Journal of Medicine* 358(4):353–361. https://doi.org/10.1056/NEJMoa071074.

Kawai, T., D. H. Sachs, M. Sykes, A. B. Cosimi, and Immune Tolerance Network. 2013. HLA-mismatched renal transplantation without maintenance immunosuppression. *The New England Journal of Medicine* 368(19):1850–1852. https://doi.org/10.1056/NEJMc1213779.

Kawamura, T., S. Miyagawa, S. Fukushima, A. Maeda, N. Kashiyama, A. Kawamura, K. Miki, K. Okita, Y. Yoshida, T. Shiina, K. Ogasawara, S. Miyagawa, K. Toda, H. Okuyama, and Y. Sawa. 2016. Cardiomyocytes derived from MHC-homozygous induced pluripotent stem cells exhibit reduced allogeneic immunogenicity in MHC-matched non-human primates. *Stem Cell Reports* 6(3):312–320.

Kehl, D., M. Generali, A. Mallone, M. Heller, A. C. Uldry, P. Cheng, B. Gantenbein, S. P. Hoerstrup, and B. Weber. 2019. Proteomic analysis of human mesenchymal stromal cell secretomes: A systematic comparison of the angiogenic potential. *NPJ Regenerative Medicine* 4:8.

Khan, A., Y. Tomita, and M. Sykes. 1996. Thymic dependence of loss of tolerance in mixed allogeneic bone marrow chimeras after depletion of donor antigen. Peripheral mechanisms do not contribute to maintenance of tolerance. *Transplantation* 62(3):380–387.

Kourtzelis, I., X. Li, I. Mitroulis, D. Grosser, T. Kajikawa, B. Wang, M. Grzybek, J. von Renesse, A. Czogalla, M. Troullinaki, A. Ferreira, C. Doreth, K. Ruppova, L. S. Chen, K. Hosur, J. H. Lim, K. J. Chung, S. Grossklaus, A. K. Tausche, L. A. B. Joosten, N. M. Moutsopoulos, B. Wielockx, A. Castrillo, M. Korostoff, U. Coskun, G. Hajishengallis, and T. Chavakis. 2019. DEL-1 promotes macrophage efferocytosis and clearance of inflammation. *Nature Immunology* 20(1):40–49.

Krampera, M., and K. Le Blanc. 2021. Mesenchymal stromal cells: Putative microenvironmental modulators become cell therapy. *Cell Stem Cell* 28(10):1708–1725.

Krishnamurthy, J., C. Torrice, M. R. Ramsey, G. I. Kovalev, K. Al-Regaiey, L. Su, and N. E. Sharpless. 2004. Ink4a/Arf expression is a biomarker of aging. *Journal of Clinical Investigation* 114(9):1299–1307.

Kurtz, J., J. Shaffer, A. Lie, N. Anosova, G. Benichou, and M. Sykes. 2004. Mechanisms of early peripheral CD4 T-cell tolerance induction by anti-CD154 monoclonal antibody and allogeneic bone marrow transplantation: Evidence for anergy and deletion but not regulatory cells. *Blood* 103(11):4336–4343.

Le Blanc, K., and D. Mougiakakos. 2012. Multipotent mesenchymal stromal cells and the innate immune system. *Nature Reviews Immunology* 12(5):383–396.

Li, Y., D. L. Hermanson, B. S. Moriarity, and D. S. Kaufman. 2018. Human iPSC-derived natural killer cells engineered with chimeric antigen receptors enhance anti-tumor activity. *Cell Stem Cell* 23(2):181–192.e185.

LoCascio, S. A., T. Morokata, M. Chittenden, F. I. Preffer, D. M. Dombkowski, G. Andreola, K. Crisalli, T. Kawai, S. L. Saidman, T. R. Spitzer, N. Tolkoff-Rubin, A. B. Cosimi, D. H. Sachs, and M. Sykes. 2010. Mixed chimerism, lymphocyte recovery, and evidence for early donor-specific unresponsiveness in patients receiving combined kidney and bone marrow transplantation to induce tolerance. *Transplantation* 90(12):1607–1615.

Looker, A. C., C.-Y. Wang. 2015. Prevalence of reduced muscle strength in older U.S. adults: United States, 2011–2012. *NCHS data brief no. 179*. Hyattsville, MD: National Center for Health Statistics.

Lu, S., J. E. Stein, D. L. Rimm, D. W. Wang, J. M. Bell, D. B. Johnson, J. A. Sosman, K. A. Schalper, R. A. Anders, H. Wang, C. Hoyt, D. M. Pardoll, L. Danilova, and J. M. Taube. 2019. Comparison of biomarker modalities for predicting response to PD-1/PD-L1 checkpoint blockade: A systematic review and meta-analysis. *JAMA Oncology* 5(8):1195–1204.

Lucas, C. M., R. J. Harris, A. Giannoudis, M. Copland, J. R. Slupsky, and R. E. Clark. 2011. Cancerous inhibitor of PP2A (CIP2A) at diagnosis of chronic myeloid leukemia is a critical determinant of disease progression. *Blood* 117(24):6660–6668.

MacKay, M., E. Afshinnekoo, J. Rub, C. Hassan, M. Khunte, N. Baskaran, B. Owens, L. Liu, G. J. Roboz, M. L. Guzman, A. M. Melnick, S. Wu, and C. E. Mason. 2020. The therapeutic landscape for cells engineered with chimeric antigen receptors. *Nature Biotechnology* 38(2):233–244.

Maekawa, T., H. Tamura, H. Domon, T. Hiyoshi, T. Isono, D. Yonezawa, N. Hayashi, N. Takahashi, K. Tabeta, T. Maeda, M. Oda, A. Ziogas, V. I. Alexaki, T. Chavakis, Y. Terao, and G. Hajishengallis. 2020. Erythromycin inhibits neutrophilic inflammation and mucosal disease by upregulating DEL-1. *Journal of Clinical Investigation Insight* 5(15): e136706.

Maher, J., R. J. Brentjens, G. Gunset, I. Rivière, and M. Sadelain. 2002. Human T-lymphocyte cytotoxicity and proliferation directed by a single chimeric TCRζ/CD28 receptor. *Nature Biotechnology* 20(1):70–75.

Markworth, J. F., L. A. Brown, E. Lim, C. Floyd, J. Larouche, J. A. Castor-Macias, K. B. Sugg, D. C. Sarver, P. C. Macpherson, C. Davis, C. A. Aguilar, K. R. Maddipati, and S. V. Brooks. 2020. Resolvin D1 supports skeletal myofiber regeneration via actions on myeloid and muscle stem cells. *Journal of Clinical Investigation Insight* 5(18):e137713.

Mauro, A. 1961. Satellite cell of skeletal muscle fibers. *Journal of Biophysical and Biochemical Cytology* 9(2):493–495.

Meizlish, M. L., R. A. Franklin, X. Zhou, and R. Medzhitov. 2021. Tissue homeostasis and inflammation. *Annual Review of Immunology* 39(1):557–581.

Menard, C., J. Dulong, D. Roulois, B. Hebraud, L. Verdiere, C. Pangault, V. Sibut, I. Bezier, N. Bescher, C. Monvoisin, M. Gadelorge, N. Bertheuil, E. Flecher, L. Casteilla, P. Collas, L. Sensebe, P. Bourin, N. Espagnolle, and K. Tarte. 2020. Integrated transcriptomic, phenotypic, and functional study reveals tissue-specific immune properties of mesenchymal stromal cells. *Stem Cells* 38(1):146–159.

Menard, C., L. Pacelli, G. Bassi, J. Dulong, F. Bifari, I. Bezier, J. Zanoncello, M. Ricciardi, M. Latour, P. Bourin, H. Schrezenmeier, L. Sensebe, K. Tarte, and M. Krampera. 2013. Clinical-grade mesenchymal stromal cells produced under various good manufacturing practice processes differ in their immunomodulatory properties: Standardization of immune quality controls. *Stem Cells and Development* 22(12):1789–1801.

Mo, F., N. Watanabe, M. K. McKenna, M. J. Hicks, M. Srinivasan, D. Gomes-Silva, E. Atilla, T. Smith, P. Ataca Atilla, R. Ma, D. Quach, H. E. Heslop, M. K. Brenner, and M. Mamonkin. 2021. Engineered off-the-shelf therapeutic T cells resist host immune rejection. *Nature Biotechnology* 39(1):56–63.

Moll, G., J. J. Alm, L. C. Davies, L. von Bahr, N. Heldring, L. Stenbeck-Funke, O. A. Hamad, R. Hinsch, L. Ignatowicz, M. Locke, H. Lonnies, J. D. Lambris, Y. Teramura, K. Nilsson-Ekdahl, B. Nilsson, and K. Le Blanc. 2014. Do cryopreserved mesenchymal stromal cells display impaired immunomodulatory and therapeutic properties? *Stem Cells* 32(9):2430–2442.

Moll, G., R. Jitschin, L. von Bahr, I. Rasmusson-Duprez, B. Sundberg, L. Lonnies, G. Elgue, K. Nilsson-Ekdahl, D. Mougiakakos, J. D. Lambris, O. Ringden, K. Le Blanc, and B. Nilsson. 2011. Mesenchymal stromal cells engage complement and complement receptor bearing innate effector cells to modulate immune responses. *PLOS ONE* 6(7):e21703.

Moll, G., I. Rasmusson-Duprez, L. von Bahr, A. M. Connolly-Andersen, G. Elgue, L. Funke, O. A. Hamad, H. Lonnies, P. U. Magnusson, J. Sanchez, Y. Teramura, K. Nilsson-Ekdahl, O. Ringden, O. Korsgren, B. Nilsson, and K. Le Blanc. 2012. Are therapeutic human mesenchymal stromal cells compatible with human blood? *Stem Cells* 30(7):1565–1574.

Moore, E. M., D. R. Maestas, C. C. Cherry, J. A. Garcia, H. Y. Comeau, L. Davenport Huyer, S. H. Kelly, A. N. Peña, R. L. Blosser, G. D. Rosson, and J. H. Elisseeff. 2021. Biomaterials direct functional B cell response in a material-specific manner. *Science Advances* 7(49):eabj5830.

Morris, H., S. DeWolf, H. Robins, B. Sprangers, S. A. LoCascio, B. A. Shonts, T. Kawai, W. Wong, S. Yang, J. Zuber, Y. Shen, and M. Sykes. 2015. Tracking donor-reactive T cells: Evidence for clonal deletion in tolerant kidney transplant patients. *Science Translational Medicine* 7(272):272ra210.

NASEM (National Academies of Sciences, Engineering, and Medicine). 2020. *Exploring novel clinical trial designs for gene-based therapies: Proceedings of a workshop*. Edited by S. Addie, M. Hackmann, J. Alper, and S. H. Beachy. Washington, DC: The National Academies Press.

NASEM. 2021. *Applying systems thinking to regenerative medicine: Proceedings of a workshop*. Edited by S. Addie, M. Hackmann, L. Teferra, A. Nicholson, and S. H. Beachy. Washington, DC: The National Academies Press.

Nikolic, B., A. Khan, and M. Sykes. 2001. Induction of tolerance by mixed chimerism with nonmyeloblative host conditioning: The importance of overcoming intrathymic alloresistance. *Biology of Blood and Marrow Transplantation* 7(3):144–153.

Norling, L. V., M. Spite, R. Yang, R. J. Flower, M. Perretti, and C. N. Serhan. 2011. Cutting edge: Humanized nano-proresolving medicines mimic inflammation-resolution and enhance wound healing. *Journal of Immunology* 186(10):5543–5547.

Palla, A. R., M. Ravichandran, Y. X. Wang, L. Alexandrova, A. V. Yang, P. Kraft, C. A. Holbrook, C. M. Schurch, A. T. V. Ho, and H. M. Blau. 2021. Inhibition of prostaglandin-degrading enzyme 15-PGDH rejuvenates aged muscle mass and strength. *Science* 371(6528).

Palmer, A. K., B. Gustafson, J. L. Kirkland, and U. Smith. 2019. Cellular senescence: At the nexus between ageing and diabetes. *Diabetologia* 62(10):1835-1841.

Passweg, J. R., P. A. Rowlings, K. A. Atkinson, A. J. Barrett, R. P. Gale, A. Gratwohl, N. Jacobsen, J. P. Klein, P. Ljungman, J. A. Russell, U. W. Schaefer, K. A. Sobocinski, J. M. Vossen, M. J. Zhang, and M. M. Horowitz. 1998. Influence of protective isolation on outcome of allogeneic bone marrow transplantation for leukemia. *Bone Marrow Transplantation* 21(12):1231–1238.

Peled, J. U., A. L. C. Gomes, S. M. Devlin, E. R. Littmann, Y. Taur, A. D. Sung, D. Weber, D. Hashimoto, A. E. Slingerland, J. B. Slingerland, M. Maloy, A. G. Clurman, C. K. Stein-Thoeringer, K. A. Markey, M. D. Docampo, M. Burgos da Silva, N. Khan, A. Gessner, J. A. Messina, K. Romero, M. V. Lew, A. Bush, L. Bohannon, D. G. Brereton, E. Fontana, L. A. Amoretti, R. J. Wright, G. K. Armijo, Y. Shono, M. Sanchez-Escamilla, N. Castillo Flores, A. Alarcon Tomas, R. J. Lin, L. Yanez San Segundo, G. L. Shah, C. Cho, M. Scordo, I. Politikos, K. Hayasaka, Y. Hasegawa, B. Gyurkocza, D. M. Ponce, J. N. Barker, M. A. Perales, S. A. Giralt, R. R. Jenq, T. Teshima, N. J. Chao, E. Holler, J. B. Xavier, E. G. Pamer, and M. R. M. van den Brink. 2020. Microbiota as predictor of mortality in allogeneic hematopoietic-cell transplantation. *The New England Journal of Medicine* 382(9):822–834.

Petersen, F. B., C. D. Buckner, R. A. Clift, N. Nelson, G. W. Counts, J. D. Meyers, and E. D. Thomas. 1987. Infectious complications in patients undergoing marrow transplantation: A prospective randomized study of the additional effect of decontamination and laminar air flow isolation among patients receiving prophylactic systemic antibiotics. *Scandinavian Journal of Infectious Diseases* 19(5):559–567.

Phelan, R., M. Arora, and M. Chen. 2020. *Current use and outcome of hematopoietic stem cell transplantation*: CIBMTR US Summary Slides.

Phillips, D., M. Matusiak, B. R. Gutierrez, S. S. Bhate, G. L. Barlow, S. Jiang, J. Demeter, K. S. Smythe, R. H. Pierce, S. P. Fling, N. Ramchurren, M. A. Cheever, Y. Goltsev, R. B. West, M. S. Khodadoust, Y. H. Kim, C. M. Schürch, and G. P. Nolan. 2021. Immune cell topography predicts response to PD-1 blockade in cutaneous T cell lymphoma. *Nature Communications* 12(1).

Raimondo, T. M., and D. J. Mooney. 2018. Functional muscle recovery with nanoparticle-directed M2 macrophage polarization in mice. *Proceedings of the National Academy of Sciences of the United States of America* 115(42):10648–10653.

Reategui, E., F. Jalali, A. H. Khankhel, E. Wong, H. Cho, J. Lee, C. N. Serhan, J. Dalli, H. Elliott, and D. Irimia. 2017. Microscale arrays for the profiling of start and stop signals coordinating human-neutrophil swarming. *Nature Biomedical Engineering* 1(7):0094.

Reynolds, G. 2017. Bring on the exercise, hold the painkillers. *The New York Times*, July 5, 2017.

Rieckmann, M., M. Delgobo, C. Gaal, L. Büchner, P. Steinau, D. Reshef, C. Gil-Cruz, E. N. T. Horst, M. Kircher, T. Reiter, K. G. Heinze, H. W. M. Niessen, P. A. J. Krijnen, A. M. Van Der Laan, J. J. Piek, J. Koch, H.-J. Wester, C. Lapa, W. R. Bauer, B. Ludewig, N. Friedman, S. Frantz, U. Hofmann, and G. C. Ramos. 2019. Myocardial infarction triggers cardioprotective antigen-specific T helper cell responses. *Journal of Clinical Investigation* 129(11):4922–4936.

Riviere, I., and M. Sadelain. 2017. Chimeric antigen receptors: A cell and gene therapy perspective. *Molecular Therapy* 25(5):1117–1124.

Russell, J. A., A. Chaudhry, K. Booth, C. Brown, R. C. Woodman, K. Valentine, D. Stewart, J. D. Ruether, B. A. Ruether, A. R. Jones, M. J. Coppes, T. Bowen, R. Anderson, M. Bouchard, L. Rallison, M. Stotts, and M. C. Poon. 2000. Early outcomes after allogeneic stem cell transplantation for leukemia and myelodysplasia without protective isolation: A 10-year experience. *Biology of Blood and Marrow Transplantation* 6(2):109–114.

Sadtler, K., K. Estrellas, B. W. Allen, M. T. Wolf, H. Fan, A. J. Tam, C. H. Patel, B. S. Luber, H. Wang, K. R. Wagner, J. D. Powell, F. Housseau, D. M. Pardoll, and J. H. Elisseeff. 2016. Developing a pro-regenerative biomaterial scaffold microenvironment requires T helper 2 cells. *Science* 352(6283):366–370.

Sadtler, K., M. T. Wolf, S. Ganguly, C. A. Moad, L. Chung, S. Majumdar, F. Housseau, D. M. Pardoll, and J. H. Elisseeff. 2019. Divergent immune responses to synthetic and biological scaffolds. *Biomaterials* 192:405–415.

Saetersmoen, M. L., Q. Hammer, B. Valamehr, D. S. Kaufman, and K. J. Malmberg. 2019. Off-the-shelf cell therapy with induced pluripotent stem cell-derived natural killer cells. *Seminars in Immunopathology* 41(1):59–68.

Savage, T. M., B. A. Shonts, A. Obradovic, S. Dewolf, S. Lau, J. Zuber, M. T. Simpson, E. Berglund, J. Fu, S. Yang, S. H. Ho, Q. Tang, L. A. Turka, Y. Shen, and M. Sykes. 2018. Early expansion of donor-specific Tregs in tolerant kidney transplant recipients. *JCI Insight* 3(22).

Schurch, C. M., S. S. Bhate, G. L. Barlow, D. J. Phillips, L. Noti, I. Zlobec, P. Chu, S. Black, J. Demeter, D. R. McIlwain, S. Kinoshita, N. Samusik, Y. Goltsev, and G. P. Nolan. 2020. Coordinated cellular neighborhoods orchestrate antitumoral immunity at the colorectal cancer invasive front. *Cell* 182(5):1341–1359 e1319.

Schwabkey, Z. I., and R. R. Jenq. 2020. Microbiome anomalies in allogeneic hematopoietic cell transplantation. *Annual Review of Medicine* 71(1):137–148.

Serhan, C. N. 2014. Pro-resolving lipid mediators are leads for resolution physiology. *Nature* 510(7503):92–101.

Serhan, C. N. 2017. Treating inflammation and infection in the 21st century: New hints from decoding resolution mediators and mechanisms. *FASEB Journal* 31(4):1273–1288.

Serhan, C. N., N. Chiang, and J. Dalli. 2015. The resolution code of acute inflammation: Novel pro-resolving lipid mediators in resolution. *Seminars in Immunology* 27(3):200–215.

Serhan, C. N., N. Chiang, and J. Dalli. 2018. New pro-resolving n-3 mediators bridge resolution of infectious inflammation to tissue regeneration. *Molecular Aspects of Medicine* 64:1–17.

Serhan, C. N., and B. D. Levy. 2018. Resolvins in inflammation: Emergence of the pro-resolving superfamily of mediators. *Journal of Clinical Investigation* 128(7):2657–2669.

Sharabi, Y., I. Aksentijevich, T. M. Sundt, 3rd, D. H. Sachs, and M. Sykes. 1990. Specific tolerance induction across a xenogeneic barrier: Production of mixed rat/mouse lympho-hematopoietic chimeras using a nonlethal preparative regimen. *Journal of Experimental Medicine* 172(1):195–202.

Sharabi, Y., and D. H. Sachs. 1989. Mixed chimerism and permanent specific transplantation tolerance induced by a nonlethal preparative regimen. *Journal of Experimental Medicine* 169(2):493–502.

Sharma, B., S. Fermanian, M. Gibson, S. Unterman, D. A. Herzka, B. Cascio, J. Coburn, A. Y. Hui, N. Marcus, G. E. Gold, and J. H. Elisseeff. 2013. Human cartilage repair with a photoreactive adhesive-hydrogel composite. *Science Translational Medicine* 5(167):167ra166.

Shin, J., T. Maekawa, T. Abe, E. Hajishengallis, K. Hosur, K. Pyaram, I. Mitroulis, T. Chavakis, and G. Hajishengallis. 2015. DEL-1 restrains osteoclastogenesis and inhibits inflammatory bone loss in nonhuman primates. *Science Translational Medicine* 7(307):307ra155.

Sierra, F., A. Caspi, R. H. Fortinsky, L. Haynes, G. J. Lithgow, T. E. Moffitt, S. J. Olshansky, D. Perry, E. Verdin, and G. A. Kuchel. 2021. Moving geroscience from the bench to clinical care and health policy. *Journal of the American Geriatrics Society* 69(9):2455–2463.

Skalak, R., and C. F. Fox. 1988. "Tissue engineering: Proceedings of a workshop, held at Granlibakken, Lake Tahoe, California, February 26–29, 1988."

Sommerfeld, S. D., C. Cherry, R. M. Schwab, L. Chung, D. R. Maestas, Jr., P. Laffont, J. E. Stein, A. Tam, S. Ganguly, F. Housseau, J. M. Taube, D. M. Pardoll, P. Cahan, and J. H. Elisseeff. 2019. Interleukin-36 -producing macrophages drive IL-17-mediated fibrosis. *Science Immunology* 4(40):eaax4783.

Sridharan, R., A. R. Cameron, D. J. Kelly, C. J. Kearney, and F. J. O'Brien. 2015. Biomaterial based modulation of macrophage polarization: A review and suggested design principles. *Materials Today* 18(6):313–325.

Stabler, C. L., J. A. Giraldo, D. M. Berman, K. M. Gattás Asfura, M. A. Willman, A. Rabassa, J. Geary, W. Diaz, N. M. Kenyon, and N. S. Kenyon. 2020. Transplantation of pegylated islets enhances therapeutic efficacy in a diabetic nonhuman primate model. *American Journal of Transplantation* 20(3):689–700.

Storb, R., R. L. Prentice, C. D. Buckner, R. A. Clift, F. Appelbaum, J. Deeg, K. Doney, J. A. Hansen, M. Mason, J. E. Sanders, J. Singer, K. M. Sullivan, R. P. Witherspoon, and E. D. Thomas. 1983. Graft-versus-host disease and survival in patients with aplastic anemia treated by marrow grafts from HLA-identical siblings. Beneficial effect of a protective environment. *The New England Journal of Medicine* 308(6):302–307.

Takeuchi, Y., H. Ito, J. Kurtz, T. Wekerle, L. Ho, and M. Sykes. 2004. Earlier low-dose TBI or DST overcomes $CD8^+$ T-cell-mediated alloresistance to allogeneic marrow in recipients of anti-CD40L. *American Journal of Transplantation* 4(1):31–40.

Themeli, M., C. C. Kloss, G. Ciriello, V. D. Fedorov, F. Perna, M. Gonen, and M. Sadelain. 2013. Generation of tumor-targeted human T lymphocytes from induced pluripotent stem cells for cancer therapy. *Nature Biotechnology* 31(10):928–933.

Tomita, Y., A. Khan, and M. Sykes. 1994. Role of intrathymic clonal deletion and peripheral anergy in transplantation tolerance induced by bone marrow transplantation in mice conditioned with a nonmyeloablative regimen. *Journal of Immunology* 153(3):1087–1098.

Tripathi, U., A. Misra, T. Tchkonia, and J. L. Kirkland. 2021. Impact of senescent cell subtypes on tissue dysfunction and repair: Importance and research questions. *Mechanisms of Ageing and Development* 198:111548.

Turner, T., M. Sok, L. Hymel, F. Pittman, W. York, Q. Mac, S. Vyshnya, H. Lim, G. Kwong, and P. Qiu. 2020. Harnessing lipid signaling pathways to target specialized pro-angiogenic neutrophil subsets for regenerative immunotherapy. *Science Advances* 6(44):eaba7702.

van Bekkum, D. W., J. Roodenburg, P. J. Heidt, and D. van der Waaij. 1974. Mitigation of secondary disease of allogeneic mouse radiation chimeras by modification of the intestinal microflora. *Journal of the National Cancer Institute* 52(2):401–404.

Van Dyke, T. E., H. Hasturk, A. Kantarci, M. O. Freire, D. Nguyen, J. Dalli, and C. N. Serhan. 2015. Proresolving nanomedicines activate bone regeneration in periodontitis. *Journal of Dental Research* 94(1):148–156.

Wagner, V., and J. Gil. 2020. T cells engineered to target senescence. *Nature* 583(7814):37–38.

Walsh, J. T., S. Hendrix, F. Boato, I. Smirnov, J. Zheng, J. R. Lukens, S. Gadani, D. Hechler, G. Gölz, K. Rosenberger, T. Kammertöns, J. Vogt, C. Vogelaar, V. Siffrin, A. Radjavi, A. Fernandez-Castaneda, A. Gaultier, R. Gold, T.-D. Kanneganti, R. Nitsch, F. Zipp, and J. Kipnis. 2015. MHCII-independent $CD4^+$ T cells protect injured CNS neurons via IL-4. *Journal of Clinical Investigation* 125(2):699–714.

Wang, D. A., S. Varghese, B. Sharma, I. Strehin, S. Fermanian, J. Gorham, D. H. Fairbrother, B. Cascio, and J. H. Elisseeff. 2007. Multifunctional chondroitin sulphate for cartilage tissue-biomaterial integration. *Nature Materials* 6(5):385–392.

Wang, H., X. Li, T. Kajikawa, J. Shin, J. H. Lim, I. Kourtzelis, K. Nagai, J. M. Korostoff, S. Grossklaus, R. Naumann, T. Chavakis, and G. Hajishengallis. 2021. Stromal cell-derived DEL-1 inhibits TFH cell activation and inflammatory arthritis. *Journal of Clinical Investigation* 131(19).

Woan, K. V., H. Kim, R. Bjordahl, Z. B. Davis, S. Gaidarova, J. Goulding, B. Hancock, S. Mahmood, R. Abujarour, H. Wang, K. Tuininga, B. Zhang, C. Y. Wu, B. Kodal, M. Khaw, L. Bendzick, P. Rogers, M. Q. Ge, G. Bonello, M. Meza, M. Felices, J. Huffman, T. Dailey, T. T. Lee, B. Walcheck, K. J. Malmberg, B. R. Blazar, Y. T. Bryceson, B. Valamehr, J. S. Miller, and F. Cichocki. 2021. Harnessing features of adaptive NK cells to generate IPSC-derived NK cells for enhanced immunotherapy. *Cell Stem Cell* 28(12):2062–2075 e2065.

Xu, M., T. Pirtskhalava, J. N. Farr, B. M. Weigand, A. K. Palmer, M. M. Weivoda, C. L. Inman, M. B. Ogrodnik, C. M. Hachfeld, D. G. Fraser, J. L. Onken, K. O. Johnson, G. C. Verzosa, L. G. P. Langhi, M. Weigl, N. Giorgadze, N. K. LeBrasseur, J. D. Miller, D. Jurk, R. J. Singh, D. B. Allison, K. Ejima, G. B. Hubbard, Y. Ikeno, H. Cubro, V. D. Garovic, X. Hou, S. J. Weroha, P. D. Robbins, L. J. Niedernhofer, S. Khosla, T. Tchkonia, and J. L. Kirkland. 2018. Senolytics improve physical function and increase lifespan in old age. *Nature Medicine* 24(8):1246–1256.

Yamazaki, M., T. Pearson, M. A. Brehm, D. M. Miller, J. A. Mangada, T. G. Markees, L. D. Shultz, J. P. Mordes, A. A. Rossini, and D. L. Greiner. 2007. Different mechanisms control peripheral and central tolerance in hematopoietic chimeric mice. *American Journal of Transplantation* 7(7):1710–1721.

Yuh, D. Y., T. Maekawa, X. Li, T. Kajikawa, K. Bdeir, T. Chavakis, and G. Hajishengallis. 2020. The secreted protein DEL-1 activates a 3 integrin-FAK-ERK1/2-RUNX2 pathway and promotes osteogenic differentiation and bone regeneration. *Journal of Biological Chemistry* 295(21):7261–7273.

Zakrzewski, J. L., M. R. van den Brink, and J. A. Hubbell. 2014. Overcoming immunological barriers in regenerative medicine. *Nature Biotechnology* 32(8):786–794.

Zhou, X., R. A. Franklin, M. Adler, J. B. Jacox, W. Bailis, J. A. Shyer, R. A. Flavell, A. Mayo, U. Alon, and R. Medzhitov. 2018. Circuit design features of a stable two-cell system. *Cell* 172(4):744–757.e717.

Zhu, H., R. H. Blum, R. Bjordahl, S. Gaidarova, P. Rogers, T. T. Lee, R. Abujarour, G. B. Bonello, J. Wu, P.-F. Tsai, J. S. Miller, B. Walcheck, B. Valamehr, and D. S. Kaufman. 2020. Pluripotent stem cell–derived NK cells with high-affinity noncleavable CD16a mediate improved antitumor activity. *Blood* 135(6):399–410.

Zhu, Y., T. Tchkonia, T. Pirtskhalava, A. C. Gower, H. Ding, N. Giorgadze, A. K. Palmer, Y. Ikeno, G. B. Hubbard, M. Lenburg, S. P. O'Hara, N. F. LaRusso, J. D. Miller, C. M. Roos, G. C. Verzosa, N. K. LeBrasseur, J. D. Wren, J. N. Farr, S. Khosla, M. B. Stout, S. J. McGowan, H. Fuhrmann-Stroissnigg, A. U. Gurkar, J. Zhao, D. Colangelo, A. Dorronsoro, Y. Y. Ling, A. S. Barghouthy, D. C. Navarro, T. Sano, P. D. Robbins, L. J. Niedernhofer, and J. L. Kirkland. 2015. The Achilles' heel of senescent cells: From transcriptome to senolytic drugs. *Aging Cell* 14(4):644–658.

Ziogas, A., T. Maekawa, J. R. Wiessner, T. T. Le, D. Sprott, M. Troullinaki, A. Neuwirth, V. Anastasopoulou, S. Grossklaus, K. J. Chung, M. Sperandio, T. Chavakis, G. Hajishengallis, and V. I. Alexaki. 2020. DHEA inhibits leukocyte recruitment through regulation of the integrin antagonist DEL-1. *Journal of Immunology* 204(5):1214–1224.

# Appendix A

# Workshop Agenda

**UNDERSTANDING THE ROLE OF THE IMMUNE SYSTEM IN IMPROVING TISSUE REGENERATION: A WORKSHOP**

November 2–3, 2021
Virtual Workshop

**TIMELINE**
November 2, 2021: 11:30 a.m.–4:30 p.m. ET
November 3, 2021: 12:00–4:00 p.m. ET

**DAY 1: NOVEMBER 2, 2021**

11:30 a.m. ET   **Welcome from the Forum Co-Chairs**

TIM COETZEE, *Forum Co-Chair*
Chief Advocacy, Services, and Science Officer
National Multiple Sclerosis Society

KATHY TSOKAS, *Forum Co-Chair*
Vice President
Regulatory, Quality, Risk Management and Drug Safety
Janssen Inc. Canada

| | |
|---|---|
| 11:40 a.m. | **Introduction and Charge to the Workshop Speakers and Participants** |

> NADYA LUMELSKY, *Workshop Planning Committee Co-Chair*
> Chief, Integrative Biology and Infectious Diseases Branch
> Program Director, Tissue Engineering and Regenerative Medicine Research Program
> National Institute of Dental and Craniofacial Research (NIDCR)
> National Institutes of Health (NIH)
>
> KIMBERLEE POTTER, *Workshop Planning Committee Co-Chair*
> Scientific Program Manager
> Biomedical Laboratory R&D Service
> Office of Research & Development
> Department of Veterans Affairs

| | |
|---|---|
| 11:50 a.m. | **Keynote: Tissue Homeostasis, Inflammation, and Repair** |

> RUSLAN MEDZHITOV
> Sterling Professor of Immunobiology
> Yale School of Medicine
> Investigator, Howard Hughes Medical Institute

| | |
|---|---|
| 12:10 p.m. | **Comment from the Patient Perspective** |

> SHERILYN GEORGE-CLINTON
> Leader
> Multiple Sclerosis: You Are Not Alone (M.S. Y.A.N.A)

## SESSION I. LESSONS LEARNED ON IMMUNE TOLERANCE AND GRAFT ACCEPTANCE

*Moderator: Sohel Talib, California Institute for Regenerative Medicine*

<u>Session Objectives</u>
- Discuss the current state of knowledge about immune tolerance mechanisms and what lessons have been learned from other areas of research, including: transplant immunology, cancer immunotherapy, maternal–fetal interface, and the microbiome.

| | |
|---|---|
| 12:20 p.m. | **Lessons Learned from Transplant Immunology**<br><br>MEGAN SYKES<br>Michael J. Friedlander Professor of Medicine and Professor of Microbiology & Immunology and Surgical Sciences (in Surgery)<br>Director, Columbia Center for Translational Immunology<br>Columbia University |
| 12:35 p.m. | **Microbiome and Immune Tolerance—If We Can't Live without It, How Best to Live with It? Lessons Learned from Allogeneic Hematopoietic Cell Transplantation**<br><br>ROBERT JENQ<br>Deputy Department Chair, Genomic Medicine<br>Associate Professor, Genomic Medicine<br>Associate Professor, Stem Cell Transplantation<br>MD Anderson Cancer Center |
| 12:50 p.m. | **Q&A with the Speakers and Participants**<br><br>Additional Panelist<br>RUSLAN MEDZHITOV<br>Sterling Professor of Immunobiology<br>Yale School of Medicine<br>Investigator, Howard Hughes Medical Institute |
| 1:25 p.m. | **Break** |

## SESSION II. ENGINEERING OF ALLOGENEIC DONOR CELLS FOR ACCEPTANCE BY THE HOST'S IMMUNE SYSTEM

*Moderator: Rachel Salzman, American Society of Gene & Cell Therapy*

Session Objectives
- Explore recent advances in engineering of allogeneic donor cells for acceptance by the host's immune system (e.g., gene editing approaches, immune silent, universal donor cells).

2:00 p.m. **Protecting Transplanted Cells from Immune Rejection Is the Key to Unlocking the Potential of Regenerative Medicine**

> SONJA SCHREPFER
> Head of Hypoimmune Platform
> Sana Biotechnology
> Adjunct Professor, Department of Surgery
> University of California, San Francisco

2:15 p.m. **Challenges to Using Mesenchymal Stem Cells in Immunomodulatory Therapies**

> KATARINA LE BLANC
> Professor of Clinical Stem Cell Research
> Karolinska Institute

2:30 p.m. **Off-the-Shelf Engineered iPSC-Derived NK and T Cells for the Treatment of Cancer**

> BOB VALAMEHR
> Chief Research and Development Officer
> Fate Therapeutics

2:45 p.m. **Q&A with the Speakers and Participants**

## SESSION III. ENDOGENOUS REGENERATION AND THE ROLE OF THE LOCAL ENVIRONMENT IN REPAIR

*Moderator: Steven Becker, National Cancer Institute*

Session Objectives
- Examine what "proper healing" looks like at the level of the local environment, and discuss relevant research gaps.
- Consider the effects of aging, gender, and other variables and pathological changes on the local environment, endogenous repair, and wound healing.

3:10 p.m. **Reversing Aging: Proinflammatory Metabolite Prostaglandin E2 Augments Muscle Regeneration**

HELEN BLAU
The Donald E. and Delia B. Baxter Foundation Professor
Director, Baxter Laboratory for Stem Cell Biology
Professor, by Courtesy, of Psychiatry and Behavioral Sciences
Stanford University

3:25 p.m. **Biomaterials for Modeling Immune Mediation in Wound Healing**

ERIKA MOORE
Rhines Rising Star Larry Hench Assistant Professor
Department of Materials Science and Engineering
University of Florida

3:40 p.m. **Endogenous Pro-Resolution and Pro-Regenerative Mechanisms in the Periodontal Tissue**

GEORGE HAJISHENGALLIS
Thomas W. Evans Centennial Professor
Department of Basic and Translational Sciences
University of Pennsylvania

3:55 p.m. **Q&A with the Speakers and Participants**

4:20 p.m. **Reflections on Day 1 and Preview of Day 2**

NADYA LUMELSKY, *Workshop Planning Committee Co-Chair*
Chief, Integrative Biology and Infectious Diseases Branch
Program Director, Tissue Engineering and Regenerative Medicine Research Program
National Institute of Dental and Craniofacial Research (NIDCR)
National Institutes of Health (NIH)

KIMBERLEE POTTER, *Workshop Planning Committee Co-Chair*
Scientific Program Manager
Biomedical Laboratory R&D Service
Office of Research & Development
Department of Veterans Affairs

4:30 p.m.  **Adjourn Workshop Day 1**

## DAY 2: NOVEMBER 3, 2021

12:00 p.m. ET  **Welcome and Overview of Day 2**

NADYA LUMELSKY, *Workshop Planning Committee Co-Chair*
Chief, Integrative Biology and Infectious Diseases Branch
Program Director, Tissue Engineering and Regenerative Medicine Research Program
National Institute of Dental and Craniofacial Research (NIDCR)
National Institutes of Health (NIH)

KIMBERLEE POTTER, *Workshop Planning Committee Co-Chair*
Scientific Program Manager
Biomedical Laboratory R&D Service
Office of Research & Development
Department of Veterans Affairs

**SESSION IV. MODULATING THE HOST IMMUNE SYSTEM TO CREATE A PRO-REGENERATION ENVIRONMENT**

*Moderator: Candace Kerr, National Institute on Aging*

Session Objectives
- Discuss the goal(s) of host immune modulation and consider what the correct molecular targets are for creating a pro-regenerative environment.

- Examine recent research advances of the role of innate and adaptive immunity in cell engraftment and endogenous tissue regeneration, and approaches for immunomodulation of the structure and function of stem cell niches for goals of tissue regeneration.

| | |
|---|---|
| 12:10 p.m. | **Cellular Senescence, Senolytics, and Organ Regeneration and Transplantation** |
| | JAMES KIRKLAND<br>Director, Robert and Arlene Kogod Center on Aging<br>Noaber Foundation Professor of Aging Research<br>Mayo Clinic |
| 12:25 p.m. | **Mapping the Immune and Tissue Environment in Healing and Non-Healing Wounds** |
| | JENNIFER ELISSEEFF<br>Jules Stein Professor, Biomedical Engineering<br>Morton Goldberg Professor, Ophthalmology<br>Professor, Materials Science & Engineering, Chemical and Biomolecular Engineering<br>Director, Translational Tissue Engineering Center<br>Johns Hopkins University |
| 12:40 p.m. | **Resolution of Acute Inflammation Stimulates Tissue Regeneration** |
| | CHARLES SERHAN<br>Endowed Distinguished Scientist & Director of the Center for Experimental Therapeutics and Reperfusion Injury<br>Brigham Women's Hospital<br>Professor of Anaesthesia<br>Harvard Medical School |
| 12:55 p.m. | **Q&A with the Speakers and Participants** |
| 1:20 p.m. | **Break** |

## SESSION V. DEVELOPING TOOLS AND PRECLINICAL MODELS FOR MONITORING AND OPTIMIZING THE HOST'S PRO-REGENERATIVE ENVIRONMENT

*Moderator: Sadik Kassim, Vor Biopharma*

Session Objectives
- Explore recent advances in monitoring and imaging of the immune system as well as the potential implications of these new approaches for clinical translation of regenerative medicines.
- Discuss challenges and opportunities with regard to preclinical models for studying the immune system involvement in response to regenerative medicine.

| | |
|---|---|
| 1:40 p.m. | **Tools for Immune Profiling and Monitoring**<br><br>GARRY NOLAN<br>Rachford and Carlota Harris Professor<br>Department of Pathology<br>Stanford University |
| 1:55 p.m. | **Engineered Immunity as a Model for Regenerative Medicine**<br><br>MICHEL SADELAIN<br>Stephen and Barbara Friedman Chair<br>Director, Center for Cell Engineering<br>Memorial Sloan Kettering Cancer Center |
| 2:10 p.m. | **Basic Immunology to Guide Regenerative Therapeutic Design**<br><br>KAITLYN SADTLER<br>Earl Stadtman Tenure-Track Investigator<br>Chief of Section on Immunoengineering<br>National Institute of Biomedical Imaging and Bioengineering |
| 2:25 p.m. | **Q&A with the Speakers and Participants** |
| 2:50 p.m. | **Break** |

## SESSION VI. FINAL PANEL: WHAT ARE SOME POSSIBILITIES TO HARNESS THE IMMUNE SYSTEM TO IMPROVE OUTCOMES FOR PATIENTS?

Session Objectives
- Explore areas of clinical therapeutic need amenable to being clinical trial candidates that could demonstrate not only proof of principle of a specific therapeutic for a clinical indication but also ways to address the immune system's role in improving tissue regeneration.

3:05 p.m.    Panel Discussion

*Moderator: Richard McFarland, Advanced Regenerative Manufacturing Institute*

Speakers:

SHERILYN GEORGE-CLINTON
Leader
Multiple Sclerosis: You Are Not Alone (M.S. Y.A.N.A)

THOMAS WYNN
Vice President, Discovery
Pfizer

EDWARD BOTCHWEY
Associate Professor
Department of Biomedical Engineering
Georgia Tech

SONJA SCHREPFER
Head of Hypoimmune Platform
Sana Biotechnology
Adjunct Professor, Department of Surgery
University of California, San Francisco

DANIELLE BROOKS
Biologist
Office of Tissues and Advanced Therapies
Division of Clinical Evaluation and Pharmacology/
  Toxicology
Center for Biologics Evaluation and Research
Food and Drug Administration

JENNIFER ELISSEEFF
Jules Stein Professor, Biomedical Engineering
Morton Goldberg Professor, Ophthalmology
Professor, Materials Science & Engineering,
  Chemical and Biomolecular Engineering
Director, Translational Tissue Engineering Center
Johns Hopkins University

3:35 p.m. **Summary of Key Points from Discussion**

RICHARD MCFARLAND
Chief Regulatory Officer
Advanced Regenerative Manufacturing Institute

3:45 p.m. **Reflections from the Workshop and Final Comments**

NADYA LUMELSKY, *Workshop Planning Committee
  Co-Chair*
Chief, Integrative Biology and Infectious Diseases
  Branch
Program Director, Tissue Engineering and Regenerative
  Medicine Research Program
National Institute of Dental and Craniofacial Research
  (NIDCR)
National Institutes of Health (NIH)

KIMBERLEE POTTER, *Workshop Planning Committee
  Co-Chair*
Scientific Program Manager
Biomedical Laboratory R&D Service
Office of Research & Development
Department of Veterans Affairs

4:00 p.m. **Adjourn Workshop Day 2**

# Appendix B

# Speaker Biographical Sketches

**Helen M. Blau, Ph.D.,** is the Donald E. and Delia B. Baxter Foundation professor and director of the Baxter Laboratory for Stem Cell Biology at Stanford University. Blau's research area is regenerative medicine with a focus on stem cells. She is world renowned for her work on nuclear reprogramming and demonstration of the plasticity of cell fate using cell fusion. Blau led the field with novel approaches to treating muscle damaged due to disease, injury, or aging. She pioneered the design of biomaterials to mimic the in vivo microenvironment and direct stem cell fate. Her laboratory discovered that transient exposure to prostaglandin E2 rejuvenates muscle stem cell function long term, enhancing muscle repair. She identified a novel hallmark of aging, the prostaglandin degrading enzyme, 15-PGDH, and showed that its inhibition augments aged muscle mass and strength. Blau served as president of the American Society for Developmental Biology, president of the International Society for Differentiation, and member of the Harvard University Board of Overseers. She is an elected member of the American Institute for Medical and Biological Engineering, the American Academy of Arts and Sciences, the American Association for the Advancement of Science, the National Academy of Medicine, and the National Academy of Sciences.

**Edward Botchwey, Ph.D.,** is an associate professor in the Wallace H. Coulter Department of Biomedical Engineering at the Georgia Institute of Technology and Emory University. His research focuses on the delivery of naturally occurring small molecules and synthetic derivatives for applications in tissue engineering and regenerative medicine. He is particularly interested in how transient control of immune response using bioactive lipids can be exploited to control trafficking of stem cells, enhance tissue vascularization, and resolve inflammation. Dr. Botchwey received both ME and Ph.D. degrees in materials science engineering and bioengineering from the University of Pennsylvania in 1998 and 2002, respectively. He was recruited to the faculty at Georgia Tech in 2012. Dr. Botchwey is a former Ph.D. fellow of the National GEM Consortium, a former postdoctoral fellow of the UNCF-Merk Science Initiative, and a recipient of the Presidential Early Career Awards for Scientists and Engineers from the National Institutes of Health. Dr. Botchwey also serves on the Board of Directors of the Biomedical Engineering Society (BMES) and serves as the secretary to the Biomedical Engineering Decade committee.

**Danielle Brooks, Ph.D.**, is a pharmacology/toxicology reviewer in the Office of Tissues and Advanced Therapies (OTAT). She received her Ph.D. in biomedical sciences with a concentration in cancer and developmental biology at the University of Tennessee Health Science Center in Memphis. Following her graduate training, Dr. Brooks completed her postdoctoral training in the Women's Malignancies Branch of the National Cancer Institute. In 2017 she joined the NCI–FDA Interagency Oncology Task Force Fellowship program as a product quality research/review fellow in the Cellular and Tissues Therapies Branch of OTAT. At the completion of her fellowship, Dr. Brooks joined the Pharmacology/Toxicology Branch, where she now focuses on the review of preclinical toxicology and pharmacology data to support the safety of cell and gene therapies, tissue-engineered products, devices, and combination products.

**Jennifer H. Elisseeff, Ph.D.**, is the Morton F. Goldberg Endowed Professor of ophthalmology and a professor of orthopaedic surgery at the Johns Hopkins School of Medicine. She is the Jules Stein Professor of ophthalmology and also holds appointments in the Johns Hopkins Department of Chemical and Biological Engineering and the Department of Materials Science and Engineering. Dr. Elisseeff is the director of the Translational Tissue Engineering Center, where she and her team of scientists are engaged in engineering technologies to repair lost tissues and are using biomaterials to develop a synthetic cornea. Dr. Elisseeff received a Ph.D. in medical engineering from the Harvard–MIT Division of Health Sciences and Technology. After doctoral studies Dr. Elisseeff was a fellow at the National Institute of General Medical Sciences Pharmacology Research Associate Program, where she worked in the National Institute of Dental and Craniofacial Research. She joined the Johns Hopkins faculty in 2001. In 2004 Elisseeff cofounded Cartilix, Inc., a startup that translated adhesive and biomaterial technologies for treating orthopedic disease, acquired by

Biomet (now Zimmer Biomet) in 2009. In 2009 she also founded Aegeria Soft Tissue and Tissue Repair, startups focused on soft tissue regeneration and wound healing. She serves on the Scientific Advisory Boards of Bausch and Lomb, Kythera Biopharmaceutical, and Cellular Bioengineering, Inc. Dr. Elisseeff has received awards including the Carnegie Mellon Young Alumni Award, the Arthritis Investigator Award from the Arthritis Foundation, and the Yasuda Award from the Society of Physical Regulation in Medicine and Biology. She was recognized by *Technology Review* magazine as a top innovator under 35 in 2002 and was included with the top 10 technologies to change the future. In 2008 Dr. Elisseeff was elected a fellow in the American Institute for Medical and Biological Engineering and a Young Global Leader in the World Economic Forum. In 2018 Dr. Elisseeff was elected to both the National Academy of Medicine and the National Academy of Engineering. She was the 2019 recipient of the NIH Director's Pioneer Award.

**Sherilyn George-Clinton** is a leader and collaborator with the Multiple Sclerosis: You Are Not Alone (M.S. Y.A.N.A) organization and a science writer for The NeuroLeadership. The NeuroLeadership is a global research organization that partners with organizations to develop their leaders and transform their cultures. Ms. George-Clinton helps create content to reach customers and prospects with the practical application of their research in performance; culture and leadership; and diversity, equity, and inclusion. As a freelance writer, Ms. George-Clinton communicates with or about patients using diverse means, working to convey technical information with nontechnical people without talking down to them and fostering engagement through storytelling. Ms. George-Clinton received her BA in English from Denison University.

**George Hajishengallis, D.D.S., Ph.D.,** earned a DDS from the University of Athens (1989) and a Ph.D. in microbiology/immunology from the University of Alabama at Birmingham (1994). He is currently the Thomas W. Evans Centennial Professor at the University of Pennsylvania, School of Dental Medicine, Department of Basic and Translational Sciences. His field of interest is the host–microbe interface, and his work has illuminated novel mechanisms of microbial dysbiosis and inflammation as well as inflammation resolution and tissue regeneration. A current focus of his laboratory involves the immunometabolic regulation of trained myelopoiesis and its effects on health and disease. He combines basic and translational research leading to innovative approaches to clinical problems, such as exemplified by periodontitis, where his preclinical work has recently led to a phase 2a clinical trial in patients with periodontal inflammation (successfully treated with a complement C3 inhibitor; AMY-101). He has published more than

210 papers (with over 24,000 citations), including in *Cell*, *Nature Immunology*, *Science Translational Medicine*, the *Journal of Clinical Investigation*, *Cell Host & Microbe*, *PNAS*, *The New England Journal of Medicine*, and *Nature Reviews Immunology*. He received the IADR Distinguished Scientist Award in Oral Biology in 2012 and the NIH/NIDCR MERIT Award in 2016. He was named Highly Cited Researcher (Clarivate/Web-of-Science) in 2018 and 2020.

**Robert Jenq, M.D.**, is the deputy department chair and an associate professor in the Department of Genomic Medicine and an associate professor in the Department of Stem Cell Transplantation at the University of Texas MD Anderson Cancer Center. His career aim is to develop and evaluate strategies that improve outcomes after hematopoietic stem cell transplantation (HSCT), in particular by augmenting graft-versus-tumor (GVT) to reduce the rates of malignant relapse and alleviating graft-versus-host disease (GVHD). To this goal, he has studied therapies that modulate alloreactive T cells in GVT and GVHD, using mouse models of HSCT. To develop strategies of augmenting antitumor immunity following HSCT, he has focused in particular on T-cell repertoire enhancement strategies. Simultaneously, he has begun to study the T-cell repertoire in the setting of GVHD. Finally, he has also examined how aspects of mucosal immunology can impact intestinal GVHD, including the microbial flora and dietary factors.

**James L. Kirkland, M.D., Ph.D.**, is the director of the Robert and Arlene Kogod Center on Aging at Mayo Clinic and Noaber Foundation Professor of Aging Research. Dr. Kirkland's research is on the contribution of fundamental aging processes, particularly cellular senescence, to age-related and chronic diseases and development of agents and strategies for targeting fundamental aging mechanisms to treat age- and chronic disease–related conditions. Additional research areas include molecular and physiological mechanisms of age-related adipose tissue and metabolic dysfunction, frailty, and loss of resilience to infections and acute diseases in old age. Dr. Kirkland's laboratory published the first article about agents that selectively eliminate senescent cells—senolytic drugs. Dr. Kirkland demonstrated that senolytic agents enhance healthspan and delay, prevent, or alleviate multiple age-related disorders and diseases in mouse models. He published the first clinical trials of senolytic drugs. He is preparing or conducting clinical studies of senolytics, including for COVID-19, frailty in elderly women, Alzheimer's disease, diabetes/obesity, osteoporosis, childhood cancer survivors, restoring function of organs from old donors to enable transplantation, idiopathic pulmonary fibrosis, preeclampsia, and others. He has more than 225 publications and holds over 50 patents. Dr. Kirkland is principal investigator of the Translational Geroscience Network (R33 AG061456), which brings together eight academic institutions to translate healthspan interventions, including senolytics and other drugs that target fundamental aging processes, from bench to bedside. He is a scientific advisory board member for several companies and academic organizations. He is president of the American Federation for Aging Research, a past member of the National Advisory Council on Aging of the National Institutes of Health, past chair of the Biological Sciences Section of the Gerontological Society of America, and past member of the Clinical Trials Advisory Panel of the National Institute on Aging. He is a board-certified specialist in internal medicine, geriatrics, and endocrinology and metabolism. Dr. Kirkland is the 2020 recipient of the Irving S. Wright Award of Distinction from the American Federation for Aging Research.

**Katarina Le Blanc, M.D., Ph.D.**, is a professor of clinical stem cell research at Karolinska Institutet. Dr. Le Blanc received her MD from the Karolinska Institutet in 1993, and her Ph.D. in 1999, also from the Karolinska Institutet. In 2002 she became a certified specialist in hematology. She has mentored many trainees, Ph.D. students, and postdocs over the years. Dr. Le Blanc has published well over 100 peer-reviewed publications and review articles, been cited more than 12,000 times, and given some 140 presentations at various national and international meetings over the last 10 years. Dr. Le Blanc's main research interest is mesenchymal stem cells, haematopoietic stem cell transplantation, and immunology. Dr. Le Blanc is a member of several international and national committees including notably the Nobel Assembly at Karolinska Institutet and The Royal Swedish Academy of Science. She is also a member of several advisory boards and has been responsible for the organization of several national and international scientific meetings, and also served on many program committees. She is the recipient of several awards including the Knut & Alice Wallenberg Foundation award for young female researchers, the Swedish Medical Society award for young scientists, and the Tobias Foundation Prize for the excellent studies of the immunological properties of mesenchymal stem cells and their use in mesenchymal stem cell therapy, awarded by the Royal Swedish Academy of Science.

**Ruslan M. Medzhitov, Ph.D.**, is the Sterling Professor of Immunobiology at Yale University School of Medicine. He is interested in understanding biological processes and phenomena from first principles. Currently, Medzhitov and his team have several areas of focus: evolutionary medicine; biology of inflammation and its relation to physiology and homeostasis; mechanisms and functions of allergy; tissue biology; non-canonical functions of the immune system; and the logic of gene expression programs.

**Erika Moore, Ph.D.**, is the Rhines Rising Star Assistant Professor in the Department of Materials Science and Engineering at the University of Florida. She earned her Ph.D. in biomedical engineering from Duke University in 2018 and her bachelor's degree in biomedical engineering from the Johns Hopkins University in 2013. Under the guidance of Dr. Jennifer L. West, Moore's doctoral thesis focused on the use of macrophages, innate immune cells, to support vascularized engineered tissue. She was awarded the Outstanding Doctoral Dissertation Award from Duke University for this work. Dr. Moore was the Provost's Postdoctoral Fellow and a visiting professor at the Johns Hopkins University in the Department of Biomedical Engineering until June 2020. Ongoing research efforts of the Moore Lab seek to understand how immune cells can be leveraged to enhance tissue regeneration, develop materials capable of directing immune cells towards desired clinical outcomes, and create in vitro tissue models to profile immune cell–blood vessel interactions in clinically relevant disease settings. Her lab is especially interested in applications for the autoimmune disorder lupus, which disproportionately affects Black women. Recently acknowledged as *Forbes* 30 Under 30 in the health care category, Dr. Moore is a former trustee on the Duke Board of Trustees. She has been awarded a KL2 NIH Training grant through the UF Clinical and Translational Science Institute, a Space Research Initiative grant, the NSF Graduate Research Fellowship, and a Ford Foundation Fellowship.

**Garry Nolan, Ph.D.**, is the Rachford and Carlota A. Harris Professor in the Department of Pathology at Stanford University School of Medicine. He trained with Leonard Herzenberg (for his Ph.D.) and Nobelist Dr. David Baltimore (for postdoctoral work for the first cloning/characterization of NF- B p65/ RelA and the development of rapid retroviral production systems). He has published over 300 research articles and is the holder of 40 U.S. patents, and has been honored as one of the top 25 inventors at Stanford University. Dr. Nolan is a member of the Parker Institute for Cancer Immunotherapy at Stanford. His areas of research include hematopoiesis, cancer and leukemia, autoimmunity and inflammation, and computational approaches for network and systems immunology. Dr. Nolan's recent efforts are focused on a single-cell analysis advance using a mass spectrometry-flow cytometry hybrid device (CyTOF) and nanoscale imaging with the "Multiparameter Ion Beam Imager" (MIBI). Further developments in imaging are enabled by CODEX—a system that inexpensively converts fluorescence scopes into high-dimensional imaging platforms. Dr. Nolan is the first recipient of the Teal Innovator Award (2012) from the Department of Defense, the first recipient of an FDA BAAA for "Bio-agent protection" from the FDA for a "Cross-Species Immune System Reference," and received the award for "Outstanding Research Achievement in 2011" from the Nature Publishing Group for his development of CyTOF applications in the immune system. Dr. Nolan is an outspoken proponent of translating public investment in basic research to serve the public welfare. He has founded or cofounded several companies (Rigel Inc., Nodality Inc., BINA, Apprise, Ionpath, Akoya.) He also serves on the boards of directors of several companies and consults for other biotechnology companies.

**Michel Sadelain, M.D., Ph.D.**, is the founding director of the Center for Cell Engineering and head of the Gene Transfer and Gene Expression Laboratory at Memorial Sloan Kettering Cancer Center, where he holds the Stephen and Barbara Friedman Chair. He is also a member of the departments of Medicine and Pediatrics at Memorial Hospital and the molecular pharmacology and chemistry program of the Sloan Kettering Institute. Dr. Sadelain's research focuses on human cell engineering and cell therapy to treat cancer and hereditary blood disorders. He and his laboratory have made major contributions to the field of chimeric antigen receptors (CARs). His group was the first to report the design of "second-generation" CARs in 2002. In addition, the Sadelain Laboratory developed artificial antigen presenting cells, auto- and trans-costimulatory engineering strategies, combinatorial antigen approaches, and inhibitory CARs; his group was first to publish dramatic molecular remissions in patients with chemorefractory acute lymphoblastic leukemia following treatment with CD19-targeted T cells.

Dr. Sadelain received his MD from the University of Paris, France, in 1984 and his Ph.D. from the University of Alberta, Canada, in 1989. After completing a clinical residency at the Centre Hospitalier Universitaire Saint-Antoine in Paris, Dr. Sadelain carried out a postdoctoral fellowship with Richard Mulligan, Ph.D., at the Whitehead Institute for Biomedical Research, Massachusetts Institute of Technology, before joining Memorial Sloan Kettering in 1994 as an assistant member. Dr. Sadelain is a member of the American Society of Cell and Gene Therapy, where he served on the board of directors from 2004 to 2007, and is an elected member of the American Society for Clinical Investigation. He has authored more than 150 scientific papers and book chapters. Dr. Sadelain holds 13 patents in immunotherapy and received the 2012 William B. Coley Award for Distinguished Research in Tumor Immunology.

**Kaitlyn Sadtler, Ph.D.**, is an Earl Stadtman Tenure-Track Investigator and the chief of the Section for Immunoengineering at the National Institute of Biomedical Imaging and Bioengineering (NIBIB) of the National Institutes of Health. Her research focuses on how the tissue microenvironment changes a host response to regenerative scaffolds used in tissue engineering and how to manipulate that environment to promote tissue growth and regeneration. Dr. Sadtler has also lent her lab's expertise to the fight against COVID-19, launching the NIH Serologic Survey to determine the number of undiagnosed infections of SARS-CoV-2 in the United States via remote blood sampling and antibody testing. Prior to beginning her lab at NIBIB, Sadtler completed a postdoctoral fellowship at the Massachusetts Institute of Technology in the Department of Chemical Engineering. There, she was awarded a Ruth L. Kirschstein Postdoctoral Fellowship for her work on immunology and tissue engineering. Dr. Sadtler was listed on BioSpace's 10 Life Science Innovators Under 40 To Watch and StemCell Tech's Six Immunologists and Science Communicators to Follow. She was recognized as a 2018 TED Fellow and delivered a TED talk that has been viewed over 2.4 million times and was listed as one of the top-viewed talks of 2018. Dr. Sadtler was selected for the 2019 *Forbes* 30 Under 30 List in Science and as a 2020 TEDMED Research Scholar. Dr. Sadtler received her Ph.D. from the Johns Hopkins University School of Medicine, where her thesis research was published in *Science* magazine, *Nature Methods*, and others.

**Sonja Schrepfer, M.D., Ph.D.,** is a professor at the University of California San Francisco (UCSF), Gladstone-UCSF Institute of Genomic Immunology, and a Scientific Founder and SVP (Head of the Hypoimmune Platform) of Sana Biotechnology, Inc. Dr. Schrepfer is the founder and director of the Transplant and Stem Cell Immunobiology (TSI) Lab. Work by Dr. Sonja Schrepfer is at the forefront of stem immunobiology and paves the way for treatment of a wide range of diseases—from supporting functional recovery of failing myocardium to the derivation of other cell types to treat diabetes, blindness, cancer, lung, neurodegenerative, and related diseases. Her work demonstrates that protecting transplanted cells from immune rejection is the key to unlocking the potential of regenerative medicine. Before pursuing a career as a research scientist, Dr. Schrepfer was trained in cardiac surgery and heart/lung transplantation and was a resident in the Cardiothoracic Surgery Departments in Munich and Hamburg, Germany. She received her Ph.D. in transplant immunology from the University of Hamburg. Dr. Schrepfer's findings have been published in leading journals such as *Nature* and *Science* and she has received numerous awards, such as the prestigious DFG-Heisenberg professorship (2009), the Innovation Award from Academia (Germany, 2014), the science award from the German Academy of Sciences (Leopoldina, 2015), and the Galenus-von-Pergamon Medal in Basic Medical Sciences (2019).

**Charles N. Serhan, Ph.D., DSc,** is the Gelman Professor at Harvard Medical School and codirector of Brigham Research Institute. His lab focuses on structural elucidation of molecules and pathways that activate resolution of inflammation. He is PI/PD of Program Project "Resolution Mechanisms in Acute Inflammation: Resolution Pharmacology" (P01-GM095467). Dr. Serhan has over 25 years of experience leading multidisciplinary research teams and led as Principle Investigator/Program Director Program (PI/PD) Project "Molecular Mechanisms in Leukocyte-Mediated Tissue Injury" (P01-DE13499) and was PI/PD for "Specialized Center for Oral Inflammation and Resolution" (P50-DE016191). Importantly, he is hands on at the bench and has trained over 60 fellows and trainees that have successful careers in academic medicine and industry.

**Megan Sykes, M.D.**, is the Michael J. Friedlander Professor of Medicine and professor of microbiology & immunology and surgical sciences (in surgery) at Columbia University. She is the founding director of the Columbia Center for Translational Immunology (CCTI) at Columbia University, director of research for the Transplant Initiative at Columbia University Medical Center (CUMC) and director of bone marrow transplantation research, Division of Hematology/Oncology at CUMC. Dr. Sykes completed her M.D. training at the University of Toronto in 1982, after which she completed a medical residency, then moved to the National Institutes of Health, Bethesda, Maryland, in 1985 as a Fogarty Visiting Associate. She joined the Massachusetts General Hospital and Harvard Medical School as an assistant professor in 1990 and was tenured as a full professor in 1999, then named to the Harold and Ellen Danser Chair in Surgery. She moved to Columbia University in 2010 to establish the CCTI, which now includes a thriving preclinical transplant program and a staff of 115 people including 19 faculty members; 16 laboratory programs in transplantation, autoimmune disease, infection, and cancer immunology; and six core facilities.

Dr. Sykes introduced the idea that graft-versus-leukemia/lymphoma effects could be separated from graft-versus-host disease (GVHD) following hematopoietic cell transplantation (HCT) by allowing GVH-reactive T cells to expand while preventing migration to the epithelial GVHD target tissues. She showed that inflammation was a critical checkpoint for such migration, which was avoided when GVH-reactive T cells were administered after conditioning-induced inflammation had subsided in mixed chimeras. These studies led to clinical trials of nonmyeloablative haploidentical HCT that achieved mixed chimerism across human leukocyte antigen (HLA) barriers without GVHD. These results paved the way for the first clinical trials of mixed chimerism that achieved renal allograft tolerance across HLA barriers. Dr. Sykes dissected the role of intrathymic and peripheral tolerance mechanisms and pioneered minimal conditioning approaches for using HCT to achieve allograft and xenograft tolerance. Her work demonstrated that (and identified mechanisms by which) mixed chimerism achieves natural antibody-producing B-cell tolerance and natural killer (NK)-cell tolerance in addition to T-cell tolerance. She developed a method of tracking the alloreactive T-cell repertoire in human transplant recipients and has used it along with other techniques to understand T-lymphocyte dynamics in the graft and the periphery of human transplant recipients. This work led to the discovery of hematopoietic progenitors in the human intestinal mucosa and demonstration of their turnover from a circulating pool in human intestinal allograft recipients. She has pioneered the development and use of humanized mouse models for the study of type 1 diabetes and for xenograft tolerance induction. Her work on xenogeneic thymic transplantation for tolerance induction led, for the first time, to long-term kidney xenograft survival in nonhuman primates.

Dr. Sykes has published more than 473 papers and chapters describing her work. She has served on the Transplantation Society (TTS) Council and has been president of the International Xenotransplantation Association (IXA) and vice president of TTS. She has received many honors and awards, including the Wyeth-Ayerst Young Investigator Award from the American Society of Transplant Physicians (1998), the AST Basic Science Established Investigator Award (2007), the TTS Roche Award for Outstanding Achievement in Transplantation Science (Basic) (2010), the TTS Award for Outstanding Achievement in Transplantation (Basic Science) (2014), and the 2018 Medawar Prize. She is a member of the Association of American Physicians, a distinguished fellow of the American Association of Immunologists, a fellow of the American Association for the Advancement of Science, and an honorary member of IXA. She was inducted into the Institute of Medicine of the National Academies (now the National Academy of Medicine) in 2009. Dr. Sykes is president-elect of the Federation of Clinical Immunology Societies (FOCIS).

**Bob Valamehr, Ph.D.**, is the chief research and development officer at Fate Therapeutics, overseeing the company's research and development activities. Previously, Dr. Valamehr has held the positions of chief development officer and vice president of cancer immunotherapy at Fate Therapeutics. Prior to that, he played key scientific roles at Amgen, the Center for Cell Control (an NIH Nanomedicine Development Center), and the Broad Stem Cell Research Center, developing novel methods to control pluripotency, to modulate stem cell fate including hematopoiesis, and to better understand cellular signaling pathways associated with cancer. He has coauthored numerous studies and patents related to stem cell biology, oncology, and materials science. Dr. Valamehr received his Ph.D. from the Department of Molecular and Medical Pharmacology at the University of California Los Angeles (UCLA), his MBA from Pepperdine University, and his BS from the Department of Chemistry and Biochemistry at UCLA.

**Thomas Wynn, Ph.D.**, is the vice president of discovery in the Inflammation and Immunology Research Unit at Pfizer and director of Pfizer's postdoctoral training program. He currently leads Pfizer's discovery efforts in the areas of immune tolerance, epithelial cell biology, immunometabolism, innate immunity, and fibrosis. Dr. Wynn is a recognized expert on immunology and fibrosis who spent 26 years at the National Institutes of Health, most recently as a senior investigator and chief of the Immunopathogenesis Section of the Laboratory of Parasitic Disease, in the National Institute of Allergy and Infectious Diseases. He received his Ph.D. from the Department of Medical Microbiology and Immunology at the University of Wisconsin in Madison, Wisconsin and has published more than 200 research papers, reviews, and book chapters in many prestigious journals such as *Nature*, *Science*, and *Nature Immunology*. Dr. Wynn has been included on the Thomson Reuters list of Highly Cited Researchers due to his important contributions to understanding the role of cytokines and growth factors in the progression and resolution of chronic inflammation, tissue regeneration, and fibrosis.

# Appendix C

# Statement of Task

The Forum on Regenerative Medicine will hold a public workshop to explore potential promising approaches to modulate the immune system and/or the regenerative medicine product for improving the clinical outcomes of tissue repair and regeneration in patients.

Workshop discussions may examine:

- lessons learned from other fields (e.g. organ or bone marrow transplantation) about the role of the host's immune system in accepting a graft to inform whether manipulation of a graft can impact the acceptance or rejection of it;
- topics such as potential approaches for modulating critical immune system pathways and communication mechanisms between the immune system and damaged and/or diseased tissues;
- the application of these lessons learned to the development and use of regenerative medicine products, for example:
  - what immune factors and pathways play a role in regeneration;
  - biomarkers that may be useful for assessing a patient's immune status or response to regenerative medicine therapies;
  - scaffolds, biomaterials, and other bioengineering tools that may modify immune responses; and
  - imaging technologies to leverage immune surveillance in patients and evaluation of the results of regenerative therapies.

A planning committee of the National Academies of Sciences, Engineering, and Medicine will organize the workshop, select and invite speakers and discussants, and moderate the discussions. Proceedings of the presentations and discussions at the workshop will be prepared by a designated rapporteur in accordance with institutional guidelines.